Case Presentations in Renal Medicine

D1394139

Other titles in preparation

Case Presentations in Cardiology

Case Presentations in Chemical Pathology

Case Presentations in Endocrinology

Case Presentations in Paediatrics

Case Presentations in Renal Medicine

R. A. Coward, MRCP
Research Fellow, Department of Renal Medicine,
Manchester Royal Infirmary

C. D. Short, MRCP
Tutor in Medicine, Department of Renal Medicine,
Manchester Royal Infirmary

N. P. Mallick, FRCP
Consultant Physician, Department of Renal Medicine,
Manchester Royal Infirmary

Butterworths
London Boston Durban Singapore Sydney Toronto Wellington

First published, 1983

© Butterworths & Co. (Publishers) Ltd 1983

British Library Cataloguing in Publication Data

Coward, R. A.
  Case presentations in renal medicine.
  —— (Case presentations)
  1. Renal insufficiency——Case studies
  I. Title   II. Short, C. D.   III. Mallick, Netar
  616.6'14   RC918.R4

  ISBN 0-407-00232-4

Library of Congress Cataloging in Publication Data

Coward, R. A.
  Case presentations in renal medicine.

  Bibliography: p.
  Includes index.
  1. Kidneys—Diseases—Case studies. I Short, C. D.
  II. Mallick, N. P.   III. Title. [DNLM: 1. Nephrology—
  Case studies. WJ 300 C874c]
  RC903.C68 1983   616.6'109   83-2802
  ISBN 0-407-00232-4

Typeset by Illustrated Arts, Sutton, Surrey
Printed and bound by Cox & Wyman Ltd., Reading

Preface

This book is primarily intended for doctors studying for higher professional examinations such as the MRCP (UK). We hope that students completing their first course in medicine will also profit from it. Our aim has been to demonstrate the way patients with renal disease present to physicians, how they are investigated and what treatment regimens may be employed. To this end we have described a variety of patients that we have encountered over the last four years, and discussed their subsequent progress. The salient features of their conditions have been highlighted. Also included towards the end of the book are some short notes on topics we felt are not dealt with satisfactorily in standard reference works.

This is neither a textbook of renal medicine, nor is it a programmed learning text, but rather a distillate of the experience of a busy nephrological centre in the UK. We would like to feel it complements the knowledge gained by SHOs and registrars working in such a unit and partially compensates for those who have not been so fortunate.

We should like to acknowledge the contribution from Dr L R Solomon who prepared the case history and discussion on the patient with hypokalaemia and the assistance and skill provided by the Department of Medical Illustration at Manchester Royal Infirmary. The encouragement and assistance, not to mention patience, on the part of Butterworth's editors was unstinting. Finally, we are pleased to thank Miss Tonie Green and Mrs Barbara Morris who have so cheerfully typed and typed again from frequently indecipherable notes.

R. A. Coward
C. D. Short
N. P. Mallick

To

Andrea Anna Mary Matthew Naomi Paula Pauline
Philippa and Stephanie

so they too may see their names in print.

Contents

Preface   **v**

Abbreviations   **x**

Approximate normal adult values   **xii**

1   Case presentations   1

  1 Urinary tract obstruction   1
  2 Polycystic disease   3
  3 Malignant hypertension   5
  4 Membranous glomerulonephritis   7
  5 Light chain disease   9
  6 Acute tubular necrosis   11
  7 Gouty nephropathy   13
  8 Focal and segmental glomerulosclerosis   15
  9 Renal artery stenosis   18
10 Leptospirosis   21
11 Pre-eclamptic toxaemia   22
12 Minimal change nephropathy   24
13 Alport's syndrome   27
14 Sub-acute bacterial endocarditis   29
15 Analgesic nephropathy   31
16 Post streptococcal glomerulonephritis   33
17 Systemic lupus erythematosus   37
18 Renal vein thrombosis   40
19 Tuberculosis   41
20 Secondary amyloidosis   44
21 Haemolytic uraemic syndrome   46
22 Mis-matched blood transfusion   48
23 Mesangial proliferative glomerulonephritis   50
24 Water intoxication   53
25 Fanconi syndrome   55
26 Diabetes mellitus   57

27 Drug induced lupus   59

28 Berger's disease   61

29 Bartter's syndrome   63

30 Primary amyloidosis   66

31 Chronic pyelonephritis   69

32 Paraquat poisoning   70

33 Goodpasture's syndrome   72

34 Medullary sponge kidney   75

35 Cystinuria   77

36 Wegener's granulomatosis   80

37 Cadmium nephropathy   82

38 Dialysis dementia   85

39 Oxalosis   87

40 Bladder tumour   89

41 Mesangiocapillary glomerulonephritis   91

42 Hyperparathyroidism   93

43 Retroperitoneal fibrosis   95

44 Prostatitis   97

45 Malaria   99

46 Benign familial haematuria   101

47 Renal osteodystrophy   103

48 Cryoglobulinaemia   106

49 Gold nephropathy   108

50 Hypernephroma   110

51 Hyperviscosity syndrome   111

52 Diabetes insipidus   113

53 Hypochloraemic alkalosis   115

54 Urethral syndrome   117

55 Interstitial nephritis   119

56 Neoplasia associated glomerulonephritis   121

57 Henoch-Schönlein syndrome   123

58 Loin pain haematuria   126

2 Topics 129

1 Examination of urine **129**
2 Creatinine clearance **132**
3 Drugs in renal disease **134**
4 Renal tubular acidosis — the acid load test **137**
5 Water deprivation/vasopressin test **139**
6 The chest x-ray in renal disease **139**
7 IVP interpretation and renal calcification **140**
8 Imaging in renal disease **142**
9 Peritoneal dialysis cannula insertion **145**
10 Continuous ambulatory peritoneal dialysis (CAPD) **147**
11 Haemodialysis **148**
12 Renal transplantation **150**
13 Nutrition and renal disease **153**
14 The face in renal disease **156**
15 Classification of glomerular diseases **157**
16 HLA and glomerular disease **159**
17 Complement and glomerular disease **161**

Index 165

Abbreviations

ACE	Angiotensin converting enzyme
ADH	Antidiuretic hormone
AFB	Acid fast bacilli
ALT	Alanine aminotransferase
ANF	Antinuclear factor
ANS	Acute nephritic syndrome
ARF	Acute renal failure
ASO titre	Anti-streptolysin 'O' titre
ATN	Acute tubular necrosis
BHS	Beta haemolytic streptococcal
CAPD	Continuous ambulatory peritoneal dialysis
CCF	Congestive cardiac failure
C_{cr}	Creatinine clearance
CIC	Circulating immune complexes
CMV	Cytomegalovirus
CRF	Chronic renal failure
CVA	Cerebrovascular accident
CXR	Chest x-ray
DI	Diabetes insipidus
DIC	Disseminated intravascular coagulation
DNA	Deoxyribonucleic acid
ECF	Extra cellular fluid
ECG	Electrocardiogram
ECV	Extra cellular volume
ERPF	Effective renal plasma flow
ESR	Erythrocyte sedimentation rate
FDP	Fibrin degradation products
FSGS	Focal and segmental glomerular sclerosis
GBM	Glomerular basement membrane
GFR	Glomerular filtration rate
GN	Glomerulonephritis
HBsAg	Hepatitis B surface antigen

x

HLA	Human lymphocyte antigen
hpf	High power field
HSS	Henoch—Schönlein syndrome
HUS	Haemolytic uraemic syndrome
IC	Immune complexes
Ig	Immunoglobulin
IMN	Idiopathic membranous nephropathy
IVP	Intravenous pyelogram
IVU	Intravenous urogram
JVP	Jugular venous pressure
KCT	Kaolin cephalin time
LFT	Liver function tests
LVF	Left ventricular failure
MCTD	Mixed connective tissue disease
MCNS	Minimal change nephrotic syndrome
MSK	Medullary sponge kidney
MSU	Midstream specimen urine
NS	Nephrotic syndrome
PAN	Polyarteritis nodosa
PAS	Para aminosalcyclic acid
PEEP	Positive end expiratory pressure
PET	Pre-eclamptic toxaemia
PFT	Pulmonary function tests
PLD	Partial lipodystrophy
PRA	Plasma renin activity
PSGN	Post streptococcal glomerulonephritis
PT	Prothrombin time
PUJ	Pelvi ureteric junction
RAS	Renal artery stenosis
RNA	Ribonucleic acid
RPGN	Rapidly progressive glomerulonephritis
RTE	Renal tubular epithelium
SAP	Serum amyloid P component
SCAT	Sheep cell agglutination test

SLE	Systemic lupus erythematosus
THC	Total haemolytic complement
TT	Thrombin time
TTP	Thrombotic thrombocytopaenic purpura
TUR	Transurethral resection
URTI	Upper respiratory tract infection
VSD	Ventricular septal defect

Approximate normal adult values

Blood	SI units	Conventional
Sodium (Na)	135–145 mmol/ℓ	135–145 mEq/ℓ
Potassium (K)	3.5–5.5 mmol/ℓ	3.5–5.5 mEq/ℓ
Chloride (Cl)	96–106 mmol/ℓ	96–106 mEq/ℓ
Bicarbonate (HCO_3)	23–29 mmol/ℓ	23–29 mEq/ℓ
Urea (Ur)	2.5–7 mmol/ℓ	15–40 mg/100 ml
Creatinine (Cr)	55–110 μmol/ℓ	0.6–1.2 mg/100 ml
Urate	0.14–0.42 mmol/ℓ males	2.25–7.0 mg/100 ml
	0.11–0.39 mmol/ℓ females	1.8–6.5 mg/100 ml
Calcium (Ca)	2.12–2.62 mmol/ℓ	9–10.5 mg/100 ml
Phosphate (PO_4)	0.8–1.4 mmol/ℓ	2.5–4.5 mg/100 ml
Total protein	60–80 g/ℓ	6–8 g/100 ml
Albumin	35–50 g/ℓ	3.5–5 g/100 ml
IgG	9.5–16.5 g/ℓ	0.95–1.65 g/100 ml
IgA	0.9–4.5 g/ℓ	0.09–0.45 g/100 ml
IgM	0.6–2.0 g/ℓ	0.06–0.2 g/100 ml

Alkaline phosphatase	20–90 IU/ℓ	3–13 King Armstrong Units/100 ℓ
Cholesterol (fasting)	3.8–7.9 mmol/ℓ males	148–305 mg/100 ml males
	4.1–8.9 mmol/ℓ females	160–350 mg/100 ml females
Complement C3 Complement C4	0.81–1.32 g/ℓ 0.25–0.62 g/ℓ	depends on method
Arterial acid base state pH 7.36–7.44		
P_{CO_2}	4.5–6.0 kPa	34–45 mmHg
P_{O_2}	12–14.7 kPa	90–110 mmHg
P_{O_2} capillary	6.7–10.7 kPa	50–80 mmHg
Bicarbonate actual	24–30 mmol/ℓ	24–30 mEq/ℓ
Base excess	−2.3–+2.3 mmol/ℓ males	
	−3.0–+1.6 mmol/ℓ females	

24 hour urine	Comment	SI units	Conventional
Volume	○□	1–3 litres	
Osmolality	○	100–1200 mosm/ℓ	
Protein (total)	×	up to 150 mg	
Albumin	×	up to 25 mg	
Calcium (Ca)	□	2.5–7.5 mmol	10.6–32 mg
Oxalate	□	0.22–0.44 mmol	10–30 mg
Cystine	++	up to 0.42 mmol	up to 38 mg
Creatinine	●	9–18 mmol	1–2 g
Phosphate	□	15–50 mmol	0.5–1.6 g
Sodium	□○	10–200 mmol	10–200 mEq
Urea	□	250–500 mmol	15–30 g
Urate	++	1–5 mmol	170–830 mg
Normetadrenaline		up to 7.0 µmol	
2 hour urine	●	< 250 000 RBC < 500 000 WBC	

Comment

×   depends on method — check with laboratory

●   males and females differ

○   dependent on fluid intake

□   dependent on dietary intake — very variable

++   dependent on endogenous metabolism, dietary intake of secondary importance

1   Case presentations

Case 1

Mr J. H.

A 64-year-old sales representative had a 25 year history of gout
diagnosed on joint aspiration. For 14 years he had been receiving
cortisone for autoimmune Addison's disease and for 7 years
thyroxine replacement therapy for myxoedema. A duodenal ulcer
was found on administering a barium meal 6 years ago and angina
had been treated with propranolol for the last 3 years.

He was admitted to hospital with a 2 month history of lethargy,
dyspnoea, ankle oedema and pruritis. There was no history of poor
urinary stream or nocturia. Clinically he was an obese 98 kg man.
Pulse was 100 and regular BP 160/95. JVP was raised 6 cm with gross
peripheral oedema, there were bilateral basal crepitations and
hepatomegaly. The bladder was not palpable and on rectal examination the prostate felt normal. Laboratory results showed urea 39.2
mmol/ℓ (235 mg/100 ml), creatinine 900 μmol/ℓ (10.2 mg/100 ml),
K 5.4 mmol/ℓ, Na 143 mmol/ℓ, Cl 100 mmol/ℓ, urate 0.50 mmol/ℓ (8.2
mg/100 ml), Hb 9 g/dl, normochromic normocytic film. Urine volume
was always more than 1ℓ/day and contained approximately 1 gram
proteinuria and 200 mmol Na/day.

Questions

1. What is the most likely diagnosis?
2. What treatment does he need?

Comment

The presumptive diagnosis was gouty nephropathy with contributory ischaemic heart disease. His condition deteriorated on high
dose diuretics and a low protein diet and he was therefore referred
for a renal opinion. The urea had risen to 54.3 mmol/ℓ (326 mg/100
ml) and creatinine to 2580 μmol/ℓ (29.2 mg/100 ml). He was
catheterized and despite lack of signs or symptoms related to
prostate obstruction there was a bladder residue of 2 litres. A brisk

diuresis of up to 8 litres a day ensued and intravenous fluids were required. One week later urea was 8 mmol/ℓ (48.1 mg/100 ml), creatinine 150 μmol/ℓ (1.69 mg/100 ml), pH 7.35 and base excess −4 with a normal acid load test. A good IVU now obtained showed prostatic obstruction. Transurethral resection of the prostate was performed and histological examination showed a localized adenocarcinoma subsequently treated by radiotherapy. Six months later urea was 7.6 mmol/ℓ (46 mg/100 ml), creatinine 100 μmol/ℓ (1.1 mg/100 ml) with a 24 hour urine volume of 2 litres.

This case illustrates uraemia with salt and water retention as the presenting feature of chronic urinary obstruction. Gross fluid overload is an unusual presenting feature in obstructive uropathy though slight oedema is well recognized. Rectal examination did not indicate prostatic enlargement but this does not exclude retrourethral prostatic enlargement with obstruction. The chronically obstructed bladder may be thin walled and easily missed on examining the obese patient.

In chronic obstructive uropathy the total exchangeable sodium is increased though this may not be reflected by oedema. Rarely a nephrogenic diabetes insipidus-like syndrome with dehydration can be the presenting feature.

Relief of obstruction can lead rapidly to a considerable improvement in renal function. The extent to which this occurs depends upon the pre-existing degree of renal damage. The consequences of acute obstruction are more readily reversible than those of the more longstanding lesion but even then, as in this case, surprisingly good results are possible. The massive diuresis following relief of obstruction reflects collectively previous salt and water retention, osmotic diuresis of urea and impaired tubular mechanisms for salt and water modulation. Thus profound extracellular fluid depletion may occur. In addition to abnormal sodium handling in the upper nephron, obstructive uropathy can cause distal tubular dysfunction with desmopressin resistant (water) diuresis and defective acidification. Unexplained renal failure in an otherwise healthy patient, at no matter what age should be investigated to exclude a reversible cause. Urinary catheterization is a quick way to exclude urethral obstruction and a high dose IVU (without dehydration) or ultrasound is advisable to assess renal size, function and pelvi-ureteric dilatation.

Case 2

Mr J. O.

In 1960, a schoolmaster, then aged 35, was noted to be hypertensive at an insurance medical but no other abnormality was revealed. His father had died at the age of 56 from a cerebrovascular accident (CVA). Two years later, his blood pressure having been controlled, he experienced several episodes of painless haematuria apparently unrelated to trauma or infection. He was then fully investigated. The pertinent finding was of polycystic disease demonstrated by intravenous urography with large kidneys, the typical 'stretched' appearance of the calyces and multiple bilateral translucent areas on the nephrogram (see p. 141).

Over the next 15 years his renal function deteriorated at a steady rate, particularly towards the latter stages. Abdominal examination at diagnosis was unremarkable but both kidneys became palpable in time. When aged 48 he experienced a right-sided hemiparesis, with sensory loss from which he made a complete recovery. His two sons were investigated in their early twenties and were also found to have polycystic kidneys. Our patient recently entered the phase of terminal renal failure and is currently being integrated into the dialysis and transplantation programme.

Questions

1. What anatomical abnormality may have been responsible for the CVA?
2. What are the implications of this disease for his children?

Comment

This man has the adult form of polycystic renal disease which is inherited as an autosomal dominant condition. Most patients have a positive family history and, although we have no proof, we suspect that his father may have had the disease. In our patient, and indeed in his father, the CVA could have been associated with the increased incidence of berry aneurysms of the Circle of Willis which is reported in adult polycystic disease. Hypertension, particularly if unrecognized or untreated, and the associated atheromatous disease could of course also have caused the CVA.

The genetic importance of this condition is that the offspring of the affected parent, who will all have a 50% chance of being affected, have frequently been born before the propositus is identified. It can be argued that these children should be investigated in their late teens and early twenties, by which time an IVU or ultrasound examination usually indicates involvement or not. They can then be informed of the risks to their own children. Computed tomography can also be employed to demonstrate the lesions.

The classification of cystic diseases of the kidney is at best arbitrary and at worst, confusing. Simple cysts are common and their significance lies in demonstrating that they are single (or a few at most) and that they are benign and not malignant. The latter is usually satisfactorily confirmed by cyst puncture, aspiration and cytological examination of the fluid obtained. Confirmation of the cystic nature of the lesion is best determined by prior ultrasonography or computed tomography.

Cystic renal lesions are also part of some rare congenital syndromes such as Turner's or tuberous sclerosis. Medullary sponge kidney and medullary cystic disease may also be considered as 'cystic' diseases of the kidney. However, the major forms are polycystic disease of infantile and adult types. In the former, which may present in the neonate or later in childhood, inheritance is autosomal recessive and results in dilatation of the distal collecting system. An associated finding of hepatic cysts and periportal fibrosis is common. Renal failure is progressive but hepatic failure is a recognized cause of death in patients with a relatively mild renal lesion.

Liver cysts are less common in the adult form, but both infantile and adult types, however, frequently have associated hypertension and haematuria. Trauma and subsequent bleeding into the kidney can be a frequent and painful problem in these patients. The rate of progression of renal failure varies from patient to patient and many years can elapse from diagnosis to the need for renal replacement therapy in adults.

The comment in the history of the steady decline in renal function refers to the observation that in many patients with progressive renal disease such as chronic pyelonephritis and glomerulonephritis, a graphical plot of the reciprocal of plasma creatinine against time frequently reveals a straight line so that the point when glomerular filtration rate will be insufficient to maintain life can be predicted fairly accurately in some cases.

Case 3

Mrs F. McG.

A 37-year-old housewife was referred from a district general hospital for further investigation and treatment of her hypertension. She gave a three month history of headaches, polyuria, polydipsia and nocturia, with haematuria for four weeks and vomiting, dizziness and blurred vision for two days. She had been on an oestrogen contraceptive pill for two years, her blood pressure being checked a year ago when it was 150/95 mmHg. During her three pregnancies she had suffered from pre-eclampsia. On admission to the referring hospital her blood pressure was 230/130 mmHg. Pulse was 110 beats per minute regular with no femoral delay. JVP was raised 2 cm and the apex beat was displaced to the anterior axillary line in the sixth intercostal space. There was a pansystolic murmur at the apex with a loud second and a third heart sound. Fundi showed bilateral papilloedema with exudates and haemorrhages. Results: Hb 10.2 g/dl, Na 120 mmol/ℓ, K 5 mmol/ℓ, urea 33 mmol/ℓ (198 mg/100 ml), creatinine 630 µmol/ℓ (7.1 mg/100 ml). There was 1 gram of proteinuria per 24 hours. Chest x-ray: enlarged heart and mild congestive changes. ECG: left ventricular hypertrophy and strain. After transfer, her blood pressure was controlled with methyldopa, hydralazine, propranolol and frusemide. Investigations for a systemic connective tissue disorder by the sheep cell agglutination test (SCAT), Latex and ANF were negative. A high dose IVU demonstrated equally poor function from both kidneys which were of normal shape but slightly reduced size. An isotope renogram showed equally poor renal function. A 24 hour urine collected prior to methyldopa treatment contained 4 µmol normetadrenaline (normal up to 7 µmol).

Questions

1. What is the definition of accelerated (malignant) hypertension?
2. What further investigations would you like to do?

Comment

This is a case of accelerated (malignant) hypertension. There is no sharp dividing line between essential and accelerated hypertension in relation to arterial pressure but rather in its effect. The pressure in the accelerated phase producing structural damage to small arteries. This is best visualized in tne fundi where exudates and haemorrhages are evidence of arteriolar damage, and is reflected in the kidney by the presence of haematuria, proteinuria and frequently a reduced creatinine clearance. A low platelet count, and raised fibrin degradation products are occasionally found in accelerated hypertension and reflect the severity of the vascular damage. A microangiopathic blood picture may occur. Hypertension with proteinuria does not imply accelerated hypertension, as a primary renal disease, such as glomerulonephritis, could give rise to both proteinuria and hypertension without causing the 'malignant' vascular damage. The presence of casts is not always helpful in identifying an underlying renal disease. Any cause of hypertension including 'essential' (idiopathic) can progess to malignant hypertension, reflecting the severity rather than the aetiology of the disease; accelerated changes are rare in aortic coarctation, Cushing's or Conn's syndromes.

The problem is to decide as in all cases of hypertension whether it is essential (primary) or secondary.

From the history and examination there is no evidence of a systemic connective tissue disease, vasculitis or coarctation of the aorta. The plasma electrolyte pattern does not suggest Conn's syndrome (primary hyperaldosteronism), where one would expect a low potassium. The normal urinary normetadrenaline is against the diagnosis of a phaeochromocytoma though catecholamine release can be intermittent. There is no evidence of intrinsic renal disease such as pyelonephritis or polycystic kidneys on the IVU although this examination does not exclude glomerulonephritis. The renogram and IVU with bilaterally poor function do not exclude an intrarenal vascular stenosis for which an arteriogram is necessary. Renin measurements have little value in diagnosing renovascular cause in accelerated hypertension as they are always high.

In this case a renal arteriogram did not show any localized arterial stenosis. The main question is therefore whether there is an underlying glomerulonephritis or if all the renal damage is secondary to the malignant hypertension. A renal biopsy was performed once the blood pressure had been controlled sufficiently to make this a safe procedure and showed normal glomeruli and tubules. There was hyalinization and thickening of the arterial walls. Immunofluorescent staining was negative.

This is therefore a case of accelerated 'essential' hypertension. Untreated the prognosis is poor with death from renal failure, heart failure or stroke within a year, however, control of blood pressure gives a much improved prognosis. Renal function may decline initially as the blood pressure is controlled because of reduced renal blood flow at the lower pressure, although once stable control is achieved the glomerular filtration rate may improve substantially.

Initially this patient required peritoneal dialysis for a week. A year later her creatinine clearance was 30 ml/minute. She eventually died four years later of intractable heart failure.

Case 4

Mr H. B.

A 64-year-old window cleaner noticed swelling of his ankles associated with a moderate increase in weight but no cardio-respiratory or other urinary symptoms. There was no previous personal or family history of renal disease. He had suffered from epilepsy from the age of 9 years (but no recent convulsions) for which he was taking phenobarbitone and phenytoin. On examination, blood pressure was 160/95 mmHg, there was bilateral pitting oedema of lower limbs up to mid-calf, but no clinical abnormality of chest, abdomen or nervous system. Rectal examination was normal.

Side room testing confirmed the presence of excessive albumin in the urine. Further investigations: Hb 13.1 g/dl, WCC $4.3 \times 10^9/\ell$, ESR 25 mm/hour, plasma urea 6.5 mmol/ℓ (39 mg/100 ml), plasma creatinine 80 μmol/ℓ (0.9 mg/100 ml), plasma albumin 31 g/ℓ, IVU and CXR normal, MSU no significant deposit, 24 hour urine protein 5 g and creatinine clearance 90 ml/minute.

This man therefore had a nephrotic syndrome and a renal biopsy showed classical changes of membranous nephropathy on light microscopy.

Questions

1. Why is a thorough clinical examination particularly necessary in this patient?
2. List some predisposing conditions associated with this pathology?
3. What is the prognosis?

Comment

The uniform thickening of the basement membrane of the peripheral capillary loops in the absence of inflammatory cells or mesangial proliferation is the hallmark of membranous nephropathy at the light microscope level, with typical 'spiking' seen on methionine—silver stain preparations. Immunofluorescent techniques show immunoglobulin and complement (usually IgG and C3 respectively) deposition in a granular fashion along the basement membrane and electron microscopy reveals the electron dense deposits to be subepithelial in position.

Patients usually present with the nephrotic syndrome, but occasionally with asymptomatic proteinuria, rarely with haematuria. Hypertension or impaired renal function may be the original clinical manifestations.

Reported series vary, but approximately 25% of adults developing the nephrotic syndrome in the UK have membranous nephropathy. The majority of patients have 'idiopathic' disease. An identical histology and clinical presentation can be secondary to lupus nephritis, occult or overt carcinoma and Hodgkin's disease, following treatment with gold or penicillamine and also in association with HbsAg, and rarely in association with light chain disease. Very occasionally a familial tendency is noted (we have 2 brothers of a sibship affected, and in another family both father and daughter have proven membranous GN). A high incidence of HLA A1, B18 and B8, and DRW3 is found in patients with idiopathic disease.

In general, treatment is aimed at controlling blood pressure, maintaining a satisfactory protein intake with sufficient but not excessive calories, and using diuretic therapy as indicated. It was believed formerly that, immunosuppresive drugs or steroids had little part to play in management, but a large prospective trial in the USA has shown that, at least in the short term steroids may delay the progress of the disease when given to subjects with normal renal function. We have witnessed some remarkably beneficial changes in patients with deteriorating renal function with high dose steroid therapy. The use of such agents however remains controversial.

Prognosis is variable: frank nephrosis is said to be of poorer prognostic significance in patients presenting to hospital; at 5 years from apparent onset about 20% are in remission, 30% have persisting proteinuria and most of the rest have nephrotic syndrome, relatively few having died. By 15 years a few of the proteinuric patients have remitted and a few have died but most of those who remained nephrotic at 5 years are either on dialysis/transplantation programmes or have died. Remission, followed by relapse, is occasionally reported, usually only after prolonged follow-up.

Currently this patient now aged 74 years is well, normotensive, has normal renal function and has been in remission for 4 years.

Case 5

Mr C. B.

Seventeen years previously a 58-year-old clerical officer had an episode of rectal bleeding caused by diverticulitis which required transfusion. Two years ago while carrying shopping and running for a bus, he experienced severe thoracic spine pain radiating around his chest to the right side. Initially he was thought to have pleurisy but the pain persisted. He was later referred to hospital and was found to have an isolated collapse of the sixth thoracic vertebrae. Skeletal survey was otherwise normal. Results showed Hb 13 g/dl, WCC $10.9 \times 10^9/\ell$ with a normal differential and an ESR of 60 mm/ hour. Urea 6.4 mmol/ℓ (38 mg/100 ml), calcium 2.3 mmol/ℓ (9.2 mg/ 100 ml). There was a polyclonal increase in immunoglobulins but no monoclonal band. Routine urine testing was normal. No specific diagnosis was made and he was treated with analgesics. Over the next two years his general health deteriorated. He had recurrent chest and ear infections. The back pain persisted, and there was a new severe pain in his right hip precipitated by movement, not occurring at night. He became dyspnoeic with no orthopnoea or paroxysmal dyspnoea. Over the last month he became increasingly thirsty but did not develop nocturia or polyuria. He was investigated in hospital. Results showed Hb 8 g/dl, WCC $15.4 \times 10^9/\ell$, normal differential, platelets $398 \times 10^9/\ell$. Normochromic normocytic film. Urea 22.4 mmol/ℓ (134 mg/100 ml), K 4.5 mmol/ℓ, creatinine 586 μmol/ℓ (6.62 mg/100 ml), Ca 3.5 mmol/ℓ (14.0 mg/100 ml), urate 0.46 mmol/ℓ (7.6 mg/100 ml). Urine was negative for protein on dipstick testing.

Questions

1. What is the probable diagnosis?
2. What tests are necessary to confirm this?
3. What is the prognosis?

Comment

Further tests showed an IgG Kappa monoclonal immunoglobulin in the serum with free Kappa light chains in the urine. Bone marrow aspiration and examination revealed 25% atypical plasma cells and skeletal survey showed extensive lytic areas in the skull and pelvis with vertebral collapse. Renal biopsy showed normal glomeruli, with no amyloid. There was however tubular atrophy with dense eosinophilic laminar tubular casts with giant cell reactions.

Intravenous fluids reduced the calcium to 3.00 mmol/ℓ (12 mg/100 ml) and on starting steroids it fell further to 2.2 mmol/ℓ (8.8 mg/100 ml). Chemotherapy with melphalan and prednisolone for the myeloma resulted in an improvement in renal function. In multiple myeloma the renal function at initial presentation is an important factor influencing prognosis and renal failure is second only to infection as a cause of death. Bence-Jones proteinuria is indicative of free immunoglobulin light chains in the urine and is present in 60–70% of patients. Light chains (mol. wt. 22 000) are normally filtered by the glomerulus and catabolized in the proximal renal tubules. The presence of urinary free light chains in myeloma or paraproteinuria is associated with renal involvement. In some cases the tubular load is greater than the catabolic capacity and therefore large amounts escape in the urine. However a number of patients continue to pass large amounts of Bence-Jones proteinuria with little or no renal damage. In the absence of glomerular damage leading to large molecular weight proteinuria the dipstick test for urinary protein will be negative despite a positive salicylsulphonic acid reaction.

On renal biopsy the myeloma kidney classically has dense intratubular casts with a giant cell, syncytial, reaction, and tubular atrophy, the degree of renal failure correlating with the extent of tubular atrophy rather than the number of casts. There may be subtle indices of renal tubular damage even when creatinine clearance is normal. This may be either proximal (aminoaciduria, renal glycosuria, hyperuricaemia and hypophosphataemia) or distal (renal tubular acidosis and lack of sensitivity to desmopressin). In treating the renal failure of myeloma it is important to rehydrate adequately, and to ensure a fluid intake of 3 litres a day if the patient can tolerate this.

Even if there is advanced renal failure some patients have recovered. It may be necessary to support patients with dialysis and to continue chemotherapy.

A renal biopsy is helpful in indicating the extent of damage. The degree of glomerular loss and tubular damage are pointers to the amount of recovery possible. The presence of amyloid is a poor prognostic sign and is often associated with the nephrotic syndrome. Amyloid occurs most frequently with Lambda light chain type but can also occur with Kappa. The mechanism of renal damage in myeloma is not fully understood. There are two main theories, first that cast formation results in blockage of tubules and, secondly, that light chains are directly nephrotoxic. Both may be correct dependent upon the circumstances of the renal failure.

Case 6

Mr M. N.

A 20-year-old policeman was admitted as an emergency at 11.45 a.m. He had been involved in a road traffic accident and was crushed underneath his motorcycle. In casualty he was conscious but pale and clammy. Blood pressure was 80/30 and pulse 130 regular. Resuscitation was begun immediately with plasma protein fraction and then whole blood. Examination revealed an extensive perineal and left loin laceration with generalized abdominal tenderness and guarding. X-rays showed a fractured pelvis with a widely separated symphysis pubis, a compound fracture of the left femur and a double fracture of the right femur, a fracture of the right radius and dislocation of the right elbow. A urinary catheter revealed fresh blood. Thomas's splints were applied to both legs and he was taken to theatre. At laparotomy a splenectomy and left nephrectomy were performed because of multiple lacerations. The perineal wound was cleaned and repaired. By the end of the operation, in the early evening, he had had 20 units of blood and 6 units of plasma protein fraction. Blood pressure was 100/80 mmHg and he was passing urine. The following morning the right foot was noted to be cold, pale and pulseless with no sensation or movement. Urine output had decreased to less than 5 ml/hour despite having maintained the central venous pressure at 8 cm. Blood tests showed K 7.4 mmol/ℓ and urea 17.4 mmol/ℓ (104 mg/100 ml). ECG showed peaked T-waves.

He was therefore referred for a renal opinion as a case of acute tubular necrosis following a period of hypotension.

12

Questions

1. What are the priorities of treatment?
2. Is the diagnosis of the renal failure correct?
3. What complications may occur?

Comment

This is a typical case of severe injury with multisystem involvement, the patient's care being shared by nephrologist, general and orthopaedic surgeons. It is therefore important to work as a team and decide upon the priorities of treatment.

The immediate life threatening factor is hyperkalaemia which is resulting in ECG abnormalities which could progress to a cardiac arrest. Hyperkalaemia is more frequent in acute rather than chronic renal failure. The rate of rise of the potassium and ECG changes are as important as the actual level in determining the urgency of treatment. The hyperkalaemia is due to the inability to remove the potassium by the kidneys in combination with the release of large amounts of intracellular potassium into the circulation from the necrotic tissue in the right leg.

Treatment of hyperkalaemia can be divided into two parts, firstly the antagonism of the cardiotoxic effects of the circulatory potassium and secondly the removal of potassium. Antagonism can be achieved by slow intravenous infusion of calcium gluconate (20–60 ml of a 10% solution under ECG monitoring), with sodium bicarbonate (100 ml 8.4%) promoting the return of potassium intracellularly. Caution should be exercised in giving sodium bicarbonate because of the large sodium load. Glucose (50 ml 50%) and insulin (25 IU soluble) together result in potassium moving into the cells and out of the circulation. These are only temporary manoeuvres and do not remove potassium from the body. This requires either haemodialysis or peritoneal dialysis. Ion exchange resins such as calcium resonium (15 g tds) given orally remove potassium but are of little value in the acute situation; however they can be used prophylactically. A retention enema of 30 to 60 g resonium in water is more effective.

In this case calcium gluconate, glucose and insulin and bicarbonate were given while preparing for haemodialysis. The potassium continued to rise with deterioration of the ECG. Haemodialysis stabilized the potassium only while it was being performed. A different approach was therefore needed — removal of the major source of potassium — the necrotic tissue in the right leg. An emergency above knee amputation resulted in adequate control of serum potassium with dialysis.

From the nephrologist's point of view the presumed diagnosis of acute tubular necrosis (ATN) secondary to haemorrhage and hypotension is the most likely cause of renal failure. However, because of the abdominal trauma damage to the remaining kidney involving the integrity of its blood supply and of urine, drainage has to be considered. It is important not to overlook urethral or ureteric obstruction as correction of this can result in rapid improvement of renal function.

Investigations for obstruction are by ultrasound, radionucleotide imaging high dose IVU and retrograde pyelography in increasing order of invasiveness. In this case ultrasound showed a normal sized kidney with no perinephric haematoma and no evidence of obstruction. Injection of contrast media demonstrated a poor nephrogram compatible with ATN but again no evidence of obstruction.

The management of established acute renal failure consists of control of hydration and electrolytes by dialysis, the provision of adequate nutrition enterally or parenterally, and the identification and treatment of infection.

Infection with *Escherichia coli*, *Pseudomonas pyocyanea* and *Streptococcus faecalis* became a major problem in this patient, originating in the perineal wound and left leg. Septicaemia with disseminated intravascular coagulation developed. Despite aggressive therapy with antibiotics, dopamine and surgical drainage the patient died ten days after his admission without regaining renal function.

An important comment is that while renal function can be substituted by by dialysis the outcome in acute renal failure is determined by the severity of the original injury or disease.

Case 7

Mr M. Y.

This 65-year-old businessman lived in East Africa. He had suffered from gout for the past 30 years. Attacks had affected particularly the first metatarsophalangeal, ankle and knee joints, but at times also the fingers and elbows. He had received symptomatic treatment only, with Butazolidin, aspirin and colchicine. Over the past 10 years, without acute symptoms, he had noticed non-fluctuant swellings around the small joints of his hands and feet and over such bony prominences as the elbows and the heels.

On a visit to England he developed an acute gastrointestinal upset, with vomiting and diarrhoea and was admitted to hospital. He had noticed weight loss of two kilograms. On examination, there were tophi over fingers, toes, elbows and ankles. Osteoarthritic changes were present in the first metatarsophalangeal joints and the knees bilaterally. Blood pressure was 170/115 mmHg, there was cardiomegaly and grade II fundal arteriolar changes.

Investigations: haemoglobin 12.0 g/dl, serum creatinine 700 μmol/ℓ, serum urea 35.0 mmol/ℓ, serum urate 0.64 mmol/ℓ, serum calcium 2.3 mmol/ℓ, creatinine clearance 10 ml/minute, urine protein 3 g/24 hour, urine urate 4.0 mmol/24 hour. Plain x-ray of the abdomen and later IVU showed small kidneys — 10.5 and 10 cm in length — with irregular margins and no calculi. The lower urinary tracts and bladder were normal. X-rays showed arthritic changes in the small joints of the feet, ankles and knees and erosive lesions in the metaphyses of joints in the feet and at the elbows.

Questions

1. What is the likely cause of the renal failure?
2. Can renal function be improved?
3. Could therapy in earlier life have averted his problems?

Comment

The renal handling of urate is very complicated. There is glomerular filtration and both tubular reabsorption and secretion. When genetically determined enzyme defects result in increased urate production, urinary excretion is increased both by filtration and secretion. In these circumstances, and particularly when the urine pH falls below 5.75, urate may precipitate and form stones. The increased filtered load of urate also results in a deposition within renal tubules and the interstitium. These deposits can be considered as broadly equivalent to those which occur in and around the joints. Urate stones and a parenchymal 'urate nephropathy' may occur separately, or with greater emphasis on one or other component. Thus, in a patient with chronic tophaceous gout, gradual impairment of renal function due to the tubulointerstitial nephropathy may occur even in the absence of urate calculi.

This is the most likely pattern of events in Mr M. Y. He had lost two kilograms in weight due to an acute gastrointestinal upset. This had resulted in extra cellular volume depletion and a further impairment of the GFR. Prerenal uraemia occurred, exacerbated by the increased protein breakdown which accompanied his illness.

His weight was restored by saline infusion, appetite improved, the gastrointestinal upset settled spontaneously and his final GFR exceeded 15 ml/minute.

Xanthine oxidase inhibitors, such as allopurinol, reduce the production of urate from hypoxanthine, the latter becoming the final metabolite in purine catabolism. Hypoxanthine is much more soluble than are urates and so does not form renal calculi. Furthermore, the excretion of urate is reduced so that the tendency to the deposition of calculi in the renal tubule is greatly diminished, and the dissolution of tophi or other urate deposits already present is promoted. Taken over a period of years, these agents would have protected Mr M. Y. from the now irreversible renal damage and extensive tophi from which he suffers. Even at the present stage of his illness, cautious use of these agents *might* delay the progression of his condition.

In this patient, chronic urate deposition was the most probable cause of the underlying renal damage. However, acute urate nephropathy may occur as a result of the chemotherapeutic treatment of haematological malignancies. As cell dissolution results, purine release is greatly increased with a consequent dramatic rise in the production of urate, which may be deposited widely. In such cases, preventative measures should include a high fluid intake and prophylactic allopurinol therapy. The urine should be kept alkaline to diminish the likelihood of urate precipitation.

The serum urate rises in patients with *chronic* renal failure from whatever cause. This does not imply that uric acid has been contributory to the renal functional impairment. Such patients, despite a raised serum urate, rarely suffer from clinical gout.

Case 8

Mrs M. P.

A 43-year-old housewife was admitted to hospital with haemoptysis and pleuritic chest pain. Further questioning elicited a history of lethargy for some months, of having noticed her ankles to be intermittently swollen and of her urine having been 'frothy' for some weeks. Just prior to presentation she had experienced an episode of severe abdominal pain, which had been self limiting. There was no history of previous renal disease, either personally or in the family, or of exposure to nephrotoxic substances.

The important findings on examination were of pitting oedema of the lower limbs extending above the knee, sacral oedema, blood pressure of 180/90 mmHg supine and 150/70 mmHg erect and the JVP was not raised. Bilateral pleural effusions were also demonstrated.

Investigations confirmed a nephrotic syndrome with a plasma albumin of 22 g/ℓ, plasma creatinine of 230 μmol/ℓ (2.6 mg/100 ml), serum cholesterol 12 mmol/ℓ, ESR 133 mm/hour and proteinuria in excess of 10 g/24 hour. No clinical, haematological, biochemical or serological evidence of myeloma, diabetes or collagenosis was found.

Renal biopsy was performed, which showed no significant light microscopic changes and the patient was therefore treated with high dose alternate day steroids in conjunction with a high protein diet. Despite an apparent diminution, proteinuria persisted at 5 g/24 hour even after eight weeks treatment. Her plasma albumin however increased to 28 g/ℓ and creatinine clearance rose from 18 ml/minute to 48 ml/minute. A further biopsy was undertaken.

Questions

1. Explain the historical features and clinical investigative findings as consequences of a glomerular lesion.
2. What is the most likely finding on the second biopsy?

Comment

The earliest symptoms of frothy urine and intermittently swollen ankles are direct consequences of proteinuria and the resultant hypoalbuminaemia. It has been recognized for a long time that not all patients experience oedema at a given plasma albumin concentration and that other factors are therefore also relevant to its production. Generally, it appears that oedema develops more readily the older the subject, possibly due in part to the greater laxity of the subcutaneous tissues. The role of natriuretic hormone in the genesis of hypoproteinaemic oedema remains speculative. Non specific tiredness is a frequent and genuine complaint of patients with hypoalbuminaemia and abdominal pain in nephrotic subjects has an undoubted pathological basis (see p. 40).

Her presenting features were those of pulmonary embolism, and while renal vein thrombosis undoubtedly occurs in nephrotic subjects it is probable that this is a secondary phenomenon in most. A thrombotic tendency certainly exists in such patients due to a combination of features including hyperfibrinogenaemia, increased circulating levels of factors V, VIII and X, low levels of the endogenous anticoagulant antithrombin III (which has a molecular weight similar to that of albumin and leaks through the glomerulus) the hyperaggregability of platelets and the hypovolaemic and haemoconcentrated state of some patients.

The clinical findings of oedema in the absence of a raised JVP, orthostatic hypotension and pleural effusions and a plasma albumin of 22 g/ℓ are self explanatory but the raised creatinine, particularly in view of the intravascular volume depletion, does not necessarily imply intrinsic renal damage. That this may at least be partly a result of hypovolaemia, and so 'pre-renal', is confirmed by the rise in creatinine clearance that occurred with the rise in plasma albumin.

Hypercholesterolaemia is an almost invariable accompaniment of the nephrotic syndrome with fasting lipid profiles of Fredrickson types IIa, IIb and IV being predominant. The explanation for these findings is uncertain but the hypoalbuminaemic state *per se* (albumin is directly involved in lipid metabolism) impaired lipid clearing mechanisms, increased lipid production and the loss, particularly if proteinuria is 'unselective', of high density lipoprotein in the urine may all contribute. The effect of these lipid abnormalities on the incidence of vascular disease in patients with glomerular disease is being debated currently.

The other specific abnormality reported in this lady is of a raised ESR. This is a direct consequence of a raised serum fibrinogen and does not necessarily imply that the underlying disease is a collagenosis, myeloma or malignancy. If remission from heavy proteinuria is obtained, the hyperfibrinogenaemia resolves and the ESR falls.

Not surprisingly, in view of the failure to respond to adequate steroid dosage, the second biopsy in this patient revealed focal segmental glomerular sclerosis (FSGS). This histopathological description is used for a fairly specific glomerular disorder, although similar appearances may be detected late in the course of otherwise typical, steroid responsive, minimal change disease, in the healing phase of a proliferative glomerulonephritis as well as in patients with Alport's syndrome. It is important to recognize that focal global sclerosis (that is the patchy loss of whole glomeruli) may occur in a variety of situations not least as a normal result of ageing.

The 'idiopathic' or 'primary' form of FSGS is usually regarded as a distinct entity. The lesions are focal (affecting some but not all glomeruli) and segmental (confined to part of the glomerulus) although global sclerosis can ensue and consist of hyaline thickening of the mesangium and capillary loops. In the course of FSGS, which affects all ages and usually presents as a nephrotic syndrome with microscopic haematuria, only the juxtamedullary glomeruli are affected initially, more superficial lesions developing later. The rest of the glomeruli are normal. Thus sampling error frequently leads to misdiagnosis in the first instance. The pathogenesis is still debated, arguments both for and against an immune complex mediated disorder or a primary vasculopathy have been proposed; IgM and C3 are usually demonstrated in the affected areas of the affected glomeruli. Interestingly, foot process fusion, the pathological hallmark of proteinurias, seems not to be restricted to the areas that are abnormal by optical and immunofluorescent techniques. In general FSGS is held to be steroid unresponsive but we have been aware of some diminution of proteinuria with high dose alternate day steroids (usually given under the misapprehension that the lesion was minimal change). Spontaneous remission is uncommon and is usually restricted to patients without a nephrotic syndrome.

The general course is of progressive renal impairment, frequently with persisting heavy proteinuria well into the terminal phases, over ten or more years. Some authorities have described a 'malignant' form of FSGS with a rapid progression to terminal renal failure within two years. Whether this represents a distinct aetiological or pathogenetic variant remains to be seen.

Case 9

Mrs B. C.

A 42-year-old housewife presented to the casualty department of the local eye hospital with a ten week history of headache, particularly worse in the evening, associated with a progressive decline in visual acuity. Her previous medical history was unremarkable. On examination, the apex beat was displaced to the anterior axillary line, there was a third heart sound with no murmurs; the JVP was normal; supine blood pressure 190/120 mmHg in both arms and the radial and femoral pulses were synchronous. There were no abdominal masses or bruits and no ankle oedema; grade III hypertensive changes were noted in the retinae. There was no clinical evidence of Cushing's syndrome or acromegaly, and no family history of renal disease or hypertension.

Results of investigations were as follows: Hb 13.1 g/dl; chest x-ray, increased cardiothoracic ratio; ECG, left ventricular hypertrophy without 'strain'; plasma urea 2.5 mmol/ℓ (15 mg/100 ml); plasma creatinine 60 μmol/ℓ (0.67 mg/100 ml); plasma potassium 3.8 mmol/ℓ; urine microscopy, no red or white cells or casts; 24 hour urine protein 0.15 g; ESR 12 mm/hour; urine normetadrenaline 3 μmol/24 hour (normal less than 7 μmol/24 hour) but an IVU demonstrated a delayed and persistent nephrogram on the right side, that kidney measuring 1.5 cm less in length than the left kidney.

Questions

1. What other test should be considered?
2. What methods could be employed to treat the hypertension?

Comment

The radiological findings are those typically, but not invariably associated with renal artery stenosis (RAS) of the right kidney. Bruits are often absent and even their presence is not diagnostic of RAS.

Treatment with a thiazide diuretic, large doses of a β-blocking drug and a peripheral vasodilator failed adequately to control the hypertension, so the possibility of surgery was considered and further investigations performed. After therapy was withdrawn, supine peripheral plasma renin activity (PRA) was 18.3 ng angiotensin II/ml/hour which is markedly raised above the normal range of 1–8 ng angiotensin II/ml/hour. An I[123] Hippuran gamma camera renogram revealed 67% and 33% function from left and right kidneys respectively from a total creatinine clearance of 80 ml/minute. For technical reasons, renal vein renin studies were not performed, but renal angiograms showed bilateral renal artery stenoses. Subsequently the right kidney was autotransplanted into the patient's right iliac fossa. Autotransplantation is a technique which involves the resiting of the affected kidney. The renal vessels can be subjected to bench surgery prior to re-implantation and this may be technically easier and more satisfactory than *in situ* excision of the stenosis and anastomosis of the refashioned ends of the renal artery, particularly if the stenosis is in a branch artery. Postoperatively a normal first circulation time of the transplanted kidney indicated satisfactory correction of the stenosis, the required dose of antihypertensive medication was substantially lower and the retinal changes reverted to normal.

Although the presence of bilateral renovascular disease may be cited as a contraindication to surgery, in this patient the operation was performed not only to improve blood pressure control but also in an attempt to preserve renal function in the transplanted kidney.

In this patient, the high PRA was compatible with renovascular hypertension, but normal values are also reported in this condition. In the later stages of the disease, hypertensive damage to the contralateral kidney may contribute to maintaining the high blood pressure. Initially, however, the rise in blood pressure is probably due to the direct pressor action of angiotensin II as evidenced by the fall in blood pressure with infusion of the angiotensin II competitive antagonist saralasin.

In the relatively simple situation of a single unilateral stenosis, divided renal vein renin studies are valuable since a better result from surgical intervention may be expected if the ratio of 'affected' to 'normal side' is greater than 1.5. It has been estimated that approximately 3% of a hypertensive population have renovascular disease and that up to 50% of these may benefit from surgery, but it must be remembered that the finding of RAS does not always imply a causal relationship, and that RAS may be found with normal blood pressure. Our patient was, typically, a young female with symptomatic hypertension due to renal artery fibromuscular dysplasia, rather than the older, usually male patient who has RAS as part of a widespread atheromatous disease. Rarely RAS may be due to external compression by tumour or other mass.

The relatively new technique of percutaneous transluminal angioplasty must be mentioned. Here, a balloon tip catheter is introduced into the stenosed segment(s) and the stenosis is dilated by inflating the balloon *in situ*.

Studies are in progress on the long term efficacy of angioplasty as compared to surgical treatment.

Finally, the development and marketing of angiotensin converting enzyme (ACE) inhibitors adds a new dimension to the specific therapy of renin driven hypertension and their value in treatment of renovascular hypertension will undoubtedly become apparent in due course.

Case 10

Mr J. L.

A 38-year-old building labourer had been unwell for two weeks with aching in the limb muscles, neck stiffness, photophobia and prolonged vomiting. He had been treated by his GP as a severe case of 'flu', with prochlorperazine, cotrimoxazole and paracetamol. His hospital admission was precipitated by a severe epistaxis. On admission he looked ill and fluid depleted. Temperature was 37.8°C, pulse 100. Blood pressure 140/85 mmHg lying, 80/60 mmHg sitting. There was a mid-systolic aortic murmur and a petechial rash on his right anterior chest wall. His conjunctivae were suffused though fundi were normal. There was no lymphadenopathy, hepatomegaly or splenomegaly. The chest was clear and neck stiffness had disappeared. Ward testing of urine was positive for blood and protein + +. Results showed Hb 13.3 g/dl, WCC 21 × 10^9/l (80% neutrophils), ESR 77 mm/hour, platelets 86 × 10^9/ℓ, coagulation tests were normal. Blood urea was 53.5 mmol/ℓ (321 mg/100 ml), Na 126 mmol/ℓ, Cl 83 mmol/ℓ, K 4.0 mmol/ℓ, bilirubin 24 μmol/ℓ (1.2 mg/100 ml), ALT 148 IU/ℓ, alk. phos. 106 IU/ℓ, ASO titre 50 Todd units. There were hyaline casts in the urine but an MSU showed no growth. Chest x-ray was normal and straight x-ray of the abdomen showed normal sized kidneys.

He was treated as having acute renal failure, due to septicaemia and disseminated intravascular coagulation, with ampicillin, cloxacillin and intravenous fluids. The temperature settled and a diuresis followed with the serum electrolytes returning to normal within seven days. Blood cultures taken on admission failed to grow any pathogen.

Questions

1. What further test would you have done?
2. What direct questions from the history would you like to ask?

Comment

This is a case of acute renal failure in a previously fit young man. Though there was evidence of a pre-renal element the casts in the urine raised the possibility of a renal lesion. Soon after admission an urgent renal biopsy was performed which showed normal glomeruli with damage to tubular cells.

In view of the history of muscle pains, meningism and epistaxis together with slightly abnormal liver function tests, leptospirosis (Weil's disease) has to be excluded. No organisms were seen either in the blood or fresh urine specimens. Blood tests however were positive with a complement fixation titre of 1:320 to leptospira icterhaemorrhagia. The renal biopsy is compatible with this diagnosis though it is occasionally diagnostic when organisms are seen in the tubular lumina. On further questioning the patient remembered cutting his hand, three weeks prior to admission on a manhole cover whilst working in rat infested sewers.

There are approximately 60 cases per year in the British Isles of leptospirosis, mostly in men because of occupational exposure. The two main types are hebdomadis, (host cattle), found in farm workers, and icterhaemorrhagia (host rats), found in builders and sewage workers. Renal damage, reflecting the severity of the infection is due to the direct tubular nephrotoxicity of the leptospira and the pre-renal dehydration secondary to vomiting. In this case the low serum sodium and chloride were due to the patient replacing the fluid lost in vomit with water rather than salt and water. Renal function usually recovers though persisting distal tubular damage is recognized. Older patients who have severe liver involvement with jaundice and also renal failure have a higher mortality. Treatment is supportive though if the diagnosis is made within five days of the infection penicillin or tetracycline may be beneficial. Leptospira are found in the blood for only a few days though they may continue to be excreted in the urine for several months. Many cases of leptospirosis, especially the hebdomadis type, are mild without kidney or liver involvement, presenting as severe 'flu' or aseptic meningitis. Leptospirosis is a notifiable disease.

Case 11

Mrs D. G.

At booking, when 11 weeks pregnant, this 19-year-old primigravid girl had a blood pressure of 115/70 mmHg with no proteinuria or urinary infection. She was in good health. Three years earlier her first cousin, then aged 23, had developed a nephrotic syndrome due to diffuse proliferative glomerulonephritis.

Pregnancy proceeded uneventfully until the 31st week when the blood pressure was 130/85 mmHg and proteinuria developed. At the 34th week the blood pressure suddenly rose to 170/110 mmHg, proteinuria reached 10 g/day and there was pitting oedema to the knees. Serum creatinine was 150 μmol/ℓ and GFR 60 ml/minute. She was treated with methyldopa and frusemide. The blood pressure fell to 160/95–105 on bed rest and there was a weight loss of two kilograms by diuresis, but fetal growth was slowed. The baby was delivered safely by Caesarean section at the 35th week.

Questions

1. What is the probable maternal diagnosis?
2. What postpartum developments may be anticipated?
3. What is the prognosis?

Comment

This is severe pre-eclamptic toxaemia (PET), of which hypertension and proteinuria are cardinal features. Oedema to this degree is unusual and a cause for some concern. The proteinuria in pre-eclampsia is mainly derived from glomerular leakage. Although it is poorly selective, it is still predominantly albumin and may be so severe that, as in this patient, a nephrotic syndrome develops.

The mechanisms involved in eclampsia and pre-eclampsia are not well defined. Such histological studies as are available suggest that, in the early stages, there is swelling of the glomerular endothelium. Severe pre-eclampsia produces profound renal cortical ischaemia, sometimes acute tubular necrosis, and rarely irreversible cortical necrosis. If accelerated hypertension supervenes, intravascular coagulation may complicate the lesion. Should DIC develop then the renal damage may be permanent. We have seen three patients in whom severe postpartum renal damage of this nature eventually led to irreversible renal failure but it must be emphasized this is a rare complication of the pre-eclamptic state.

The plasma volume is reduced in pre-eclampsia and this too contributes to renal impairment.

Once the baby has been delivered the probability is that however severe, the maternal abnormalities will remit completely but this may take several weeks. So the approach is to deliver the baby as soon as feasible to give both mother and baby the best opportunity of avoiding problems. If delivery is delayed, fetal death may result, the placenta being compromised by the mother's cardiovascular state. During this time the mother must be protected from the still potentially dangerous effects of the acute pathophysiology by dietary control of salt and protein intake, hypotensive therapy and diuretics. Eclamptic fits which are thought to be related to cerebral oedema and hypertension remain a hazard during the immediate postpartum period and blood pressure and fluid balance must be carefully monitored. In this patient the family history of glomerular disease was not relevant. The heavy proteinuria is quite consistent with the pre-eclamptic state.

Three months postpartum the blood pressure was 120/70 mmHg, the GFR was greater than 100 ml/minute and there was no proteinuria. All therapy had been withdrawn. Mrs D. G. was told that further pregnancy would probably be uneventful but that, statistically, it was more likely that problems of hypertension and proteinuria would recur in her than in someone who had had an entirely uncomplicated first pregnancy.

The choice of hypotensive drug is important. Methyldopa is the traditional agent, since it does not appear to compromise the placenta or influence fetal development. Hydralazine has been favoured, its vasodilator properties being held to benefit placental integrity. Theoretically β-blocking drugs may promote premature uterine contraction, but in practice they can be very effective in pregnancy and their use should be considered when difficulty arises in obtaining control with other agents. It is safer for both mother and baby that the blood pressure is controlled than that a potent drug be withheld.

Diuretic therapy should be reserved for treating fluid retention. Both thiazide drugs (insulin antagonism) and frusemide (nerve deafness) have side effects which may be manifested in the fetus, but not at the usual dose levels.

Case 12

Mr W. R.

A 17-year-old schoolboy developed ankle and periorbital swelling. The oedema spread rapidly to involve the whole of his legs and abdomen, and his weight increased by 10 kg. He had presented at the age of 5 with generalized oedema and proteinuria, and had been treated with prednisolone which induced a prompt remission. Frequent relapses over the next two years led to him receiving a course of cyclophosphamide (2.5 mg/kg daily for 8 weeks) following which the proteinuria abated for 4 years. Subsequently he had yearly relapses, usually beginning during springtime, and each one being steroid sensitive.

On this occasion there was marked oedema of legs, genitalia, sacrum and abdominal wall with clinical evidence of ascites and bilateral pleural effusions, the latter being confirmed radiologically. Other investigations revealed: Hb 13.3 g/dl, ESR 70 mm/hour, collagen screen negative, plasma albumin 20 g/ℓ, plasma creatinine 60 μmol/ℓ (0.7 mg/100 ml), with a creatinine clearance in excess of 100 ml/minute, 24 hour urine protein excretion 19 g, fibrinogen 681 mg/100 ml (normal 200–400), selectivity index 0.10.

Questions

1. What is the diagnosis and what are the characteristic findings of the renal biopsy on optical and electron microscopy and immunofluorescence?
2. What are the usual treatment regimens employed?

Comment

Renal biopsy in this patient revealed only a mild increase in mesangial cells and matrix but no other histological abnormality except for total (global) sclerosis of one of the 25 glomeruli examined. Immunofluorescence using antisera against immunoglobulins and complement components was negative and electron micrographs showed no detectable electron dense deposits (immune complexes) but did demonstrate the fusion of the foot processes (podocytes) of the epithelial cells lining the urinary space, which is found in all cases of glomerular proteinuria, not only in 'minimal change nephropathy' (MCN). These immunofluorescent and ultrastructural findings are typical of MCN, the appearances under the light microscope are usually normal or at most show slight mesangial cell proliferation and matrix expansion.

MCN is steroid sensitive, and failure to respond to adequate doses of prednisolone is an indication for rebiopsy which then usually reveals a glomerular lesion such as focal segmental glomerular sclerosis (FSGS) or frank mesangial proliferation with obvious immunoglobulin and complement deposition by immuno-fluorescence, which had not been apparent on the original biopsy. This patient was treated with 100 mg of prednisolone (1–1.5 mg/kg or 60 mg/m^2) on alternate days, which resulted in disappearance of the proteinuria in two weeks and the dose was then decreased by 10 mg/week. If proteinuria does not respond promptly, steroid therapy may be continued for up to 8 weeks at the original dose. In practice, most subjects go into remission much sooner than this. The well-known side effects of steroid therapy are less frequent on alternate day regimens.

Cyclophosphamide is reserved for patients who relapse frequently or who appear to be steroid dependent. Prolonged and sometimes permanent remission is usually obtained. The original problems encountered following the use of this alkylating agent, such as sterility, do not appear to be significant if a schedule of 2.5 mg/kg/day for a maximum of 8 weeks is adhered to. The course of cyclophosphamide may be given concurrently with the decreasing dose of prednisolone. Because cyclophosphamide may induce marrow toxicity, white cell and platelet counts should be checked, preferably each week. There is no evidence that with this regimen, cyclophosphamide induces carcinogenesis, but the potency of such immunosuppressive drugs in inducing serious side effects must be kept in mind.

Highly selective proteinuria as measured by the ratio of clearances of IgG to transferrin, is a common feature of MCN but this is not diagnostic, and may be found in other glomerulopathies.

MCN is the diagnosis in about 90% of the 30 per million children (mainly males and usually between the ages of 2 and 5 years) who develop nephrotic syndrome each year in the UK. Many of these children have one or two episodes of proteinuria which then appears to go into permanent remission, although some become chronic and frequent relapsers. It is a clinical impression that there is an increased incidence of atopy in the children affected (and/or their first degree relatives). There is an association of the disease with HLA DR7. It is less common in adults, with males and females equally affected, accounting for at most 25% of the 10 per million population per year of adults who develop nephrotic syndrome (NS). Very rarely it may be associated with underlying malignancy, usually Hodgkin's disease, and the proteinuria remits with treatment of the lymphoproliferative disorder.

There is some debate as to whether MCN, which itself does not progress to chronic renal failure, may develop into another glomerulopathy such as FSGS and so proceed to renal impairment. This discussion stems from problems in histopathological interpretation. It is best to consider MCN, with minimal histological changes and response to steroids, as having a good prognosis. Before the advent of antibiotics, infection, commonly pneumococcal peritonitis, was a serious cause of morbidity and mortality. It must be remembered that an impaired GFR in a patient presenting with NS is consistent with a diagnosis of MCN, since the abrupt appearance of massive proteinuria and rapid development of gross oedema, both of which seem to occur with greater frequency in MCN as opposed to the other glomerulopathies, can lead to a significant pre-renal element consequent upon a low plasma albumin. Such hypovolaemia may even result in ATN. With remission of the MCN, renal function is restored to normal.

Case 13

Mr J. S.

A 20-year-old rubber worker had nerve deafness from birth. His mother was a deaf mute and two of his sisters had hearing impairments.

At the age of 16 he presented to his general practitioner with a 4 year history of enuresis. A urine specimen showed protein and blood on dipstick testing, and he was referred for a urological opinion where haematuria was confirmed with 30–40 red blood cells per high power field. Chest x-ray and intravenous urogram (IVU) were normal. No biochemical tests were performed and cystoscopy revealed no abnormality.

There was no relief of symptoms with Tofranil (imipramine) or Cetiprin, and he was lost to follow-up.

He presented again three years later complaining of epistaxis, headaches, nausea, lethargy and dyspnoea. On examination he was clinically anaemic. Pulse was 80/minute regular. Blood pressure 200/120 mmHg in both arms. The apex was displaced to the sixth intercostal space in the anterior axillary line. There was a triple rhythm with a loud aortic second sound and a systolic ejection murmur. Chest was clear. Fundi showed severe arteriovenous nipping and silver wiring. Anterior lenticonus was present.

Results showed Na 138 mmol/ℓ, K 4.9 mmol/ℓ, urea 74.6 mmol/ℓ

(448 mg/100 ml), creatinine 1670 μmol/ℓ (18.9 mg/100 ml), calcium 1.42 mmol/ℓ, PO$_4$ greater than 3.0 mmol/ℓ, alkaline phosphatase 62 IU/ℓ, albumin 33 g/ℓ. Haemoglobin 5.0 g/dl, WBC 4.7 × 10^9/ℓ, platelets 94 × 10^9/ℓ, ESR 142 mm/hour. ECG: left ventricular hypertrophy with 'strain'. The chest x-ray: enlarged heart with clear lung fields. IVU: smooth kidneys reduced in size from the previous examination, with bilaterally equally poor concentration of dye.

Questions

1. What is the diagnosis?
2. What is the inheritance?

Comment

Renal biopsy showed an end stage sclerosed kidney compatible with the diagnosis of Alport's syndrome (hereditary chronic nephritis). Alport drew attention to the association of hereditary nephritis with nerve deafness in 1927. The clinical and pathological features have been variable in different series. Microscopic haematuria can occur in affected infants of under a year. The haematuria may become macroscopic following upper respiratory tract infections or exercise. Frequency, nocturia and hypertension develop during adolescence. The nephrotic syndrome, (occurring in 20% of cases) can precede progressive renal failure.

Ocular involvement occurs in 10% of patients. The usual finding is anterior lenticonus which is clinically detected when observing the red reflex with an ophthalmoscope at a distance of about one metre from the eye. There appears to be a central dense cataract, which disappears on approaching the eye. Macular lesions and atrophy of the iris have also been reported.

The disease is more severe in males. Nephritis and deafness can occur independently in the same family. Individuals with nerve deafness may have children with renal disease and vice versa. The inheritance is that of an autosomal dominant with higher 'penetrance' in males, and occurs in all races.

Histologically the characteristic lesion is the electron microscope finding of a focally thickened glomerular basement membrane with areas of extreme thinning. Foam cells containing cholesterol and its esters are also found in tubules and glomeruli, with progressive atrophy. Immunofluorescence is negative.

There is no specific therapy. There is no evidence of recurrence in transplanted kidneys.

It is always important when taking a history in renal disease to ask about deafness or eye problems in other members of the family as well as in the patient.

Case 14

Mrs G. A.

A 24-year-old divorcee was admitted as an emergency. At the age of 5 she was found to have a heart murmur. Her first pregnancy, aged 20 was uneventful, and during her second pregnancy, aged 21, she was seen by a cardiologist but no specific treatment was needed. However, at 32 weeks' gestation she became hypertensive, with normal renal function and was admitted until delivery (with forceps at 39 weeks) of a normal baby. At the age of 22 she had had an uneventful termination of pregnancy at 10 weeks' gestation followed by insertion of an IUD. Eight months prior to admission she had a gonococcal urethral discharge treated with ampicillin and probenecid. Her present illness began one week before admission with generalized aches and pains in the muscles, nausea, epistaxis and loose motions. She became confused, aggressive and was hallucinating. Temperature was 40.5°C with a pulse of 120 beats/minute. Blood pressure 140/90 lying and standing. There was a triple rhythm and a harsh systolic murmur at the left sternal edge. There was no evidence of vasculitis and the fundi were normal. The spleen was just palpable. Routine ward testing of urine showed protein +++, blood +++. Urgent results were, Hb 13.1 g/dl, WCC $11.4 \times 10^9/\ell$ (85% neutrophils), platelets $40 \times 10^9/\ell$, FDP 1:16 (normal 1:8), urea 10 mmol/ℓ (60 mg/100 ml). Chest x-ray was normal.

The following day her urine output was 300 ml and plasma urea had risen to 20 mmol/ℓ (120 mg/100 ml). Her breathing had become distressed and arterial blood gases showed a pH 7.2, P_{O_2} 40 and P_{CO_2} 50 mmHg.

Questions

1. What is the diagnosis?

2. What is the mechanism of the renal injury?
3. What is the treatment?

Comment

This is a young girl with a known heart murmur. During her second pregnancy the diagnosis of a ventricular septal defect (VSD) was made but as she was asymptomatic the only advice given then was to ensure antibiotic cover for any instrumentation.

Her presentation is that of an acute bacterial infection (pyrexia, neutrophilia and splenomegaly). A septic abortion with *Clostridium welchii* was excluded by history, examination and culture. Blood cultures taken on admission grew *Staphylococcus aureus*. The diagnosis was acute staphylococcal bacterial endocarditis on the VSD. Her dyspnoea and hypoxaemia would support this as serial chest x-rays showed diffuse shadowing progressing to cavitation, due to blood borne spread into the lung of septic emboli from the right side of the heart.

Her renal failure was acute in onset. On admission her urea was only slightly raised at 10 mmol/ (60 mg/100 ml) but she had large amounts of protein and blood in her urine. There are several causes of uraemia in septicaemia. Excess fluid losses due to pyrexia, and poor fluid intake due to debility cause desalination and hypovolaemic shock, which may progress to acute tubular necrosis (ATN). Septic endotoxic shock with disseminated intravascular coagulation can result in altered renal blood flow and ATN. Circulating immune complexes may become deposited in the glomerulus causing a glomerulonephritis. Often there is a combination of these factors, and administration of nephrotoxic drugs (e.g. gentamicin) in inappropriate doses can exacerbate the renal damage.

In this case the blood pressure was normal with no postural hypotension thus excluding significant blood volume depletion. The low platelet count and slightly raised FDPs suggest mild disseminated intravascular coagulation (DIC). Bacterial infections have been implicated in immune complex glomerulonephritis. In bacterial endocarditis very high levels of circulating soluble immune complexes have been found. These complexes can deposit in the kidney causing glomerulonephritis and also in arterial walls causing a vasculitis. The Janeway spots and splinter haemorrhages of bacterial endocarditis are due to a vasculitis of small arterioles and not septic emboli as was previously thought. There was no evidence of immune complexes causing a systemic vasculitis in this patient.

It is important to take blood cultures on the suspicion of infection before starting antibiotic treatment. There is little benefit from taking more than three pairs of cultures or timing the culture to coincide with spikes of temperature and no difference between arterial and venous blood. Once the cultures are taken treatment should not be delayed whilst awaiting results. It is best to start with a broad spectrum high dose regimen such as gentamicin and penicillin or a cephalosporin, changing treatment to more specific agents when the organism and sensitivity are known.

In this case treatment on admission was with cefoxitin changing to flucloxacillin and vancomycin when the organism was identified. The IUD was removed as a possible nidus of infection but was sterile on culture. The renal failure progressed and the patient required haemodialysis within 4 days of admission. The major problem however was the respiratory failure. Assisted ventilation was necessary within 2 days of admission using high concentrations of oxygen and positive end expiratory pressure (PEEP) to maintain oxygenation. As a complication she developed several pneumothoraces and eventually died from respiratory failure 2 weeks after admission without recovering renal function.

At post mortem there was a small VSD with vegetations on the right side only. In the lungs there were multiple abscesses.

The kidneys showed changes of acute tubular necrosis with little glomerular damage.

Case 15

Mr H. T.

A 54-year-old clergyman initially presented as an urgency to casualty 6 years ago having fainted whilst taking a service. He was slow to recover from this collapse and was admitted to hospital for observation. Systemic enquiry revealed a 5 year history of daily frontal headaches which were worse during periods of tension. He was normotensive and had no focal neurological signs. Results however showed a blood urea of 45 mmol/ℓ (270 mg/100 ml), creatinine 530 μmol/ℓ (6 mg/100 ml) with a creatinine clearance of 8 ml/minute. Proteinuria, 1 g/24 hour, MSU had 100 WBC/high power field and 50 RBC/high power field with no growth. An intravenous urogram was reported as showing bilaterally small, poorly functioning scarred kidneys. There was no evidence of tuberculosis.

A diagnosis of chronic renal failure secondary to pyelonephritis was made and he was treated with a Giovenetti diet which reduced the blood urea to 15 mmol/ℓ (90 mg/100 ml).

Two years later he had an episode of haematuria with loin pain and passed what he thought was a small blood clot. At this time his blood pressure was raised at 180/110 mmHg and he was treated with methyl dopa.

Following a slow decline in renal function to a clearance of 6 ml/minute three unsuccessful attempts were made to establish an arteriovenous fistula. These failures were thought to be due to depletion of extracellular fluid volume. Despite severe renal failure and hypertension, he appeared to waste salt, being unable to reduce sodium excretion to below 120 mmol/day.

Questions

1. Are you happy with the diagnosis of pyelonephritis?
2. What questions would you like to ask the patient?

Comment

No adequate diagnosis has been made here apart from chronic renal failure with small irregular kidneys — the presumed diagnosis being pyelonephritis. At this level of renal function with a protracted history renal biopsy is unlikely to be helpful, only showing 'end stage' sclerosed kidney.

There are two main clues in the history. The episode of haematuria with a clot, and a salt losing state with poor renal function.

'Salt losing nephritis' with chronic renal failure is rare and implies either obstructive renal failure or a rare complication of such tubulo-interstitial renal diseases as pyelonephritis, myeloma, analgesic nephropathy, polycystic disease or heavy metal poisoning.

Pyelonephritis and glomerulonephritis do not cause haematuria severe enough to produce a clot. Was it really a clot? On close questioning he was sure that it was not a stone. Because of its fleshy and pale colour, this 'clot' could be a sloughed papilla. Papillary necrosis and shedding is due to medullary ischaemia and may occur in diabetes, analgesic nephropathy, sickle cell disease, tuberculosis and macroglobulinaemia.

The IVU was reviewed and although the calyceal detail was poor there was distortion and destruction of the papillae with typical ring shadows (p. 141).

With this information the patient was questioned about his analgesic intake. He admitted that for the past 11 years he had taken two or three compound analgesic headache tablets or powders almost every day.

Analgesic nephropathy was first recognized in Swiss watch makers in 1953 and since then has been increasingly diagnosed as a major, but treatable, cause of renal damage. In Australia it is said to account for 25% of chronic renal failure and in UK at least 10%. Typically it occurs in middle aged women presenting with chronic renal failure though there may be an acute presentation as renal colic due to a sloughed papilla, haematuria, urinary infection or hypertension. These patients may have a previous psychiatric history though the analgesics may be taken for genuine musculoskeletal pain or headaches or just as 'tonics'. Patients may deny analgesic consumption and informed relatives may have to be questioned to obtain an accurate history. Half the patients have recurrent urinary tract infections, although even when the urine is sterile there is an increased excretion of white and red cells. Impaired distal tubular function may be the first sign of renal damage. Most patients are salt losers but despite this hypertension is common (10–50%). Early diagnosis is important as stopping analgesic consumption may halt the progression of the disease.

The analgesic drugs involved are usually compounds containing phenacetin and either paracetamol or aspirin (e.g. Anadin, Codis, Beechams powders, Codeine Co or Veganin), although the formulation of these compounds has now been changed and phenacetin is no longer available 'over the counter'. Most patients have consumed 3–20 kg of drugs over 5–30 years though living in a hot climate with consequent dehydration can reduce these figures. A complication of analgesic nephropathy is the development of transitional cell carcinoma of the renal pelvis.

With adequate saline repletion our patient had a successful A-V fistula constructed though he received a transplant before it was needed.

Case 16

Miss K. J.

A 13-year-old schoolgirl was noticed by her parents to have periorbital swelling. Ten days earlier, she had complained to her general practitioner of a sore throat and had received a one week course of penicillin-V 250 mg orally qds. She returned to her doctor, and on direct questioning admitted to having passed only small quantities of urine during the previous 48 hours.

On examination periorbital oedema was confirmed, the jugular venous pressure was raised and blood pressure was 150/95 mmHg supine. Dipstick testing of her urine revealed the presence of blood and protein and she was referred to the local hospital for further investigation and management.

Questions

1. What is the clinical diagnosis?
2. How may this be confirmed?
3. What is the most likely pathological diagnosis?

Comment

This presentation is of an acute nephritic syndrome (ANS). This is a clinical diagnosis, with a combination of oliguria, fluid retention with oedema, raised blood pressure and evidence of circulatory overload. Urinalysis shows haematuria (which may be microscopic or macroscopic) in the presence of proteinuria (frequently only + or ++ on dipstick testing). Urine microscopy revealed the presence of granular and red cell casts in the deposit.

The history of a sore throat one to three weeks earlier, and treatment with penicillin, suggests that a beta haemolytic streptococcal (BHS) infection may have been responsible. In this particular case the girl's general practitioner had taken a throat swab at the original presentation which had grown just such an organism. The delay from original infection to clinical manifestation of renal disorder is typical of such an illness, by which time, particularly if antibiotics have been given, the throat swab culture may be negative. Serological confirmation is then sought by looking for a raised antistreptolysin O titre (ASO titre). In one celebrated study, in only 30% of children presenting with an ANS could evidence of a recent streptococcal infection be demonstrated. There are a number of reports implicating other agents as being responsible for an ANS including *Streptococcus viridans* (endocarditis), mumps, Coxsackie B and Epstein-Barr virus infections, and a similar clinical presentation may occur in multisystem diseases including systemic lupus and the Henoch–Schönlein syndrome in the absence of preceding infection.

Haematuria developing within hours or days of an upper respiratory tract infection (URTI) is more suggestive of Berger's disease.

Post streptococcal glomerulonephritis (PSGN) is the best documented of the postinfectious nephritides. Only certain phage types of Lancefield Group A organisms are nephritogenic. Unlike in our patient, however, it usually occurs in children just starting school. Most series report boys being affected twice as commonly as girls. All ages, however, may be affected.

The clinical manifestations in this patient were typical but not all need to be present when glomerular damage has occurred. One careful prospective study of adults presenting with URTI which were proven to be due to BHS has shown that many subclinical cases of glomerulonephritis occur which are only detected by examination of the urine. All of these subjects who were biopsied had a proliferative glomerulonephritis. They all underwent spontaneous resolution. In clinical cases the latent period from sore throat (or occasionally BHS sepsis elsewhere, such as skin) to nephritis, the frequent finding of a low serum C3 level (which usually recovers by the eighth week) and the characteristic histopathological changes in the glomeruli, all point to an immunological pathogenesis. In the acute phase, the usual (but not invariable) finding on renal biopsy is a diffuse proliferative glomerulonephritis, that is, all glomeruli examined show an increase in mesangial cells and matrix with endothelial cell proliferation and infiltration by neutrophils of both the capillaries and mesangium. Occasionally epithelial crescents may be present. The characteristic immunofluorescent pattern is of IgG and C3 deposition in a granular fashion along the glomerular basement membrane (GBM) and in the mesangium. Some very recent evidence suggests that a BHS antigen may be demonstrated by immunofluorescence in biopsy tissue. The hallmark of this lesion is the finding of subepithelial humps (which, by implication, are aggregations of immune complexes) demonstrated on electron microscopy. However, such subepithelial 'humps' may also be found in other glomerulopathies, and in diffuse proliferative glomerulonephritis electron dense deposits may also be found in other areas including the mesangium and subepithelial sites. If a repeat biopsy is taken in children or adults some weeks or months later, it may show a picture similar to mesangial proliferative glomerulonephritis, the 'aggressive' proliferative phase having resolved.

The course and prognosis of patients with PSGN and diffuse proliferative change histologically is still not completely clear. What is apparent is that in the vast majority of subjects complete recovery ensues. In many patients a few days of oliguria, with a transient rise in serum creatinine, is followed by a diuretic phase. Biochemical normality is quickly restored and urine abnormalities disappear, although microscopic haematuria and gradually decreasing proteinuria may persist for many years. In very few patients, irreversible renal failure may develop virtually at onset. In others, progressive decline takes place over a few months, and in another group chronic renal failure appears after many years. Current experience, however, indicates that children fare much better than adults.

The long-term course and prognosis of patients with PSGN which was subclinical in the first instance is not known. It could be reasonable to expect a benign outcome, but the subsequent development of hypertension (in the absence of urinary abnormalities) or of chronic renal failure with 'small kidneys', cannot be excluded.

Treatment is non-specific. In the acute phase, providing hypertension, hyperkalaemia and fluid overload are appropriately controlled, the condition is usually self-limiting. The development of hypertensive encephalopathy or life-threatening hyperkalaemia of course needs more aggressive intervention. Antibiotics are indicated in a patient who has not been so treated, and some authorities also recommend antibiotics for asymptomatic BHS carriers, for example, family members. Dialysis in the acute phase is possibly only infrequently required. Once oliguria is prolonged, however, the probability of full recovery lessens and long-term renal replacement therapy may become essential. The value of long-term follow-up in these patients is contested. One of the most surprising features of this disease is its apparent decrease in incidence in the UK over the last few years. And one of the least understood problems in PSGN is the exact mechanism of development of oliguria. It was thought that endothelial swelling led to capillary lumen obliteration and, hence, an effective fall in GFR: this does not appear, though, to be the whole story.

Our patient had a diuresis soon after admission having been mildly azotaemic. No specific therapy was required but moderate proteinuria did persist at about 2–3 g/24 hours for some years. By the sixth year of follow-up she was in complete remission. She remains well and normotensive. Interestingly, she now has half-normal levels of the serum complement component C4. Whether this was the case before her nephritis is unknown and the pathogenetic implications thereof remain purely speculative.

Case 17

Miss E. B.

A 15-year-old schoolgirl with no significant previous medical or surgical history developed pain and swelling of her ankle joints, and soon after had signs and symptoms of an inflammatory arthritis involving fingers, wrists, elbows and knees. These symptoms persisted for some weeks until she became breathless and a chest x-ray revealed a pleural effusion, cytological examination of the aspirate showing typical SLE cells. Proteinuria was also demonstrated and a creatinine clearance of 30 ml/minute was recorded. Prednisolone, 40 mg daily, and a thiazide diuretic were commenced and she was transferred for consideration of renal biopsy after three weeks' treatment. At that time, there was no rash, oedema or lymphadenopathy and no detectable abnormalities on abdominal examination or in the respiratory, cardiovascular or neurological systems, save for a blood pressure of 180/110 mmHg both supine and erect. The following results were obtained: Hb 8.8 g/dl; ESR 42 mm/hour; plasma albumin 28 g/ℓ; plasma urea 8.6 mmol/ℓ (52 mg/100 ml); plasma creatinine 50 μmol/ℓ (0.57 mg/100 ml), rheumatoid factor not detected; SLE cells, present; ANF positive + +; anti DNA antibodies 46 units/ml (normal < 10 units/ml); 24 hour urine protein 10–12 g; creatinine clearance 112 ml/minute; platelets 406 × 10^9/ℓ; C3 120 mg/100 ml (normal 100–200 mg/100 ml); C1q and C4 both reduced at 34% and 24% of normal respectively; urine microscopy, granular casts present; circulating C1q binding IgG complex levels were raised; direct Coombs test, negative. Renal biopsy was performed. She was treated with a high protein diet, propranolol and azathioprine 125 mg daily added to her regimen. The malaise and arthritis present at the onset of her illness soon disappeared and 2 years after presentation the proteinuria had fallen to less than 1 g in 24 hours, creatinine clearance was 120 ml/minute with a plasma creatinine of 60 μmol/ℓ (0.7 mg/100 ml), ANF had become negative but anti-ds DNA antibody was still present at 14 units/ml, complement components were normal except for a persistently low C4 level. She is maintained on prednisolone 5 mg on alternate days and azathioprine 75 mg daily, and the hypertension, which commonly develops in association with lupus nephritis, has remitted.

Question

1. What histological appearances of the glomeruli are consistent with the diagnosis?

Comment

Systemic lupus erythematosus (SLE) is primarily a disease of young and middle aged women. It is estimated that in excess of 70% develop a renal lesion which may be asymptomatic and only manifested by proteinuria and microscopic haematuria, or a nephrotic syndrome or acute glomerulonephritis may develop. They may be present at clinical onset or appear at any time, even years later. Nephropathy may be part of the generalized lupus process. It is becoming recognized that glomerular disease with histological features consistent with SLE and positive serological findings only, may be present in the absence of other systemic features. Furthermore, there are reports of abnormal biopsy findings in the presence of normal urinalysis, urine microscopy and renal function. It must be remembered that LE cells are present in less than 80% of patients with otherwise typical SLE; that ANF is present in 95% of such patients but is also positive in a substantial proportion of normal subjects as well as individuals with other 'connective tissue' diseases. Currently the serum concentration of antibody to double stranded DNA (anti-ds DNA) is used as a diagnostic marker and also as an indicator of disease activity. For the latter purpose a change in value rather than any absolute level may be more significant.

The nephritis of SLE results from the deposition or *in situ* formation of immune complexes (IC) within the glomerulus and is mediated by activation of the complement cascade, usually via the classical pathway. The significance of type, size and concentration of circulating IC on pathogenesis and prognosis is unknown.

A variety of histopathological findings are observed in lupus patients, from mild mesangial proliferation to severe diffuse proliferative and crescentic lesions, and including abnormalities identical to those found in idiopathic membranous nephropathy and, occasionally, a mixed picture with features of both membranous and proliferative change. No biopsy appearance is pathognomonic for SLE but the presence of a variety of immunoglobulins and complement components demonstrated on immunofluorescence, or the detection of deposits in tubular basement membrane in an otherwise idiopathic membranous lesion, does indicate the need to consider lupus as a diagnosis.

The prognosis of patients with membranous change is said to parallel that of the idiopathic variety. The results from early series suggested a worse prognosis with the more severely proliferative lesions, but more recent evidence indicates that this is not necessarily the case. Whether or not this is due to treatment (predominantly with steroids) is unclear. It has certainly become apparent that 'innocent' looking biopsy appearances may 'transform' to more severe ones, and that the reverse may also occur, sometimes apparently in response to treatment. The contention that a nephrotic syndrome conferred a worse prognosis has been challenged.

More confusion is present in regard to therapy. It appears that little benefit is gained in treatment of the more benign, mild lesions, but steroid therapy may help some patients with more aggressive disease. The original enthusiasm for combination therapy with the addition of azathioprine or cyclophosphamide to the steroid has been blunted, with recent data indicating little or no benefit. Intermittent 'pulse therapy' (methylprednisolone 1 g i.v. for 3–5 days) to treat exacerbations of the disease with relatively low dose maintenance therapy may be beneficial as may plasmaphaeresis in certain, as yet poorly defined, situations.

For patients as a whole certain serological tests do show correlations with other measures of disease, e.g. changes in GFR, but these same trends do not necessarily apply to the individual. Interpretation of complement levels is difficult. C3 and C4 levels are often low. This may be due to consumption or decreased production and in rare cases inherited deficiencies of Clq, C4 and C2 predispose to the development of a lupus like syndrome, interestingly usually without anti-ds DNA being detectable. No single satisfactory indication of long-term prognosis has yet been demonstrated.

Claims for therapeutic benefit should be interpreted with caution since some patients improve spontaneously and remain in prolonged and even permanent remission but as yet the overall prognosis of lupus nephropathy is still poor. Relapse following apparent complete remission is documented. Terminal renal failure can now be treated with dialysis and transplantation and recurrent disease in a transplanted kidney has been infrequently reported.

The role of viruses as aetiological agents of this disease in man is unproven, but a genetic predisposition is implied by the increased frequency of the HLA antigens B8, DRW2 and DRW3 in affected individuals.

Case 18

Mr M. C.

A 32-year-old draughtsman complained of increasing swelling of his legs over a 6 week period and was admitted for investigation. He had been very well prior to this with no previous serious illnesses.

On examination he was pyrexial, at 38 °C, and had gross bilateral pitting oedema to the waist. His JVP was low with blood pressure falling from 160/90 mmHg lying to 150/70 mmHg standing. His chest was dull at the right base with reduced air entry.

Laboratory investigations showed: a plasma albumin of 19 g/ℓ, with 10 g/day proteinuria. Urea 14 mmol/ℓ (84 mg/100 ml). Creatinine 200 μmol/ℓ (2.3 mg/100 ml). Hb 15 g/dl, WCC 14 × 10^9/ℓ (85% neutrophils), platelets 175 × 10^9/ℓ. Chest x-ray showed a right pleural effusion the protein content of which was 5 g/ℓ.

A diagnosis of nephrotic syndrome was made but before any treatment was instituted he complained of severe pain in the right iliac fossa, with tenderness. Bowel sounds were normal as was an x-ray of the abdomen.

Questions

1. What is the differential diagnosis?
2. What management do you recommend?

Comment

This is a case of abdominal pain in a patient with severe nephrotic syndrome. The first hurdle in establishing a diagnosis is to decide if the two are related. Any cause of acute abdomen has to be considered. The most likely with this history and findings is appendicitis. He underwent laparotomy. The appendix was normal, the right kidney was enlarged. Isotope renography demonstrated diminished right renal clearance of [131]I Hippuran. On ultrasound examination there was no pulsation of the right renal vein which had a reduced internal diameter. The diagnosis was confirmed by inferior vena caval venography where there was lack of 'streaming' on the right side because of a right renal vein thrombosis.

Renal vein thrombosis may complicate a severe nephrotic syndrome, but is rarely a cause. The reason for this complication is the tendency to hypercoagulability which results when fibrinogen, factor VIII and factor IX levels are high (characteristic findings in the nephrotic syndrome) while plasminogen activation and the anti-thrombin III level are reduced. Biopsy and angiographic studies suggest that, initially, thrombosis involves the renal venules and extends from there to the larger veins. Any form of glomerular pathology may be present, but membranous nephropathy is the most frequent reported finding in association with renal vein thrombosis.

The reported incidence of asymptomatic occlusion of the renal venules ranges from 2 to 30%. Occlusion of the major renal veins is rare but may be sudden, as in this case, with engorgement and even infarction of the kidney. Only in such cases is there evidence of global renal impairment. Treatment may be by fibrinolysis, anti-coagulants or surgical thrombectomy. The last is of limited value since only the major veins can be cleared. Prompt medical treatment can promote complete resolution as happened in this patient with heparin. His nephrotic syndrome later remitted spontaneously.

The acute abdomen in nephrotic syndrome occurs particularly in young (adolescent) subjects with severe proteinuria (> 10 g/day) and plasma albumin < 20 g/ℓ. Apart from renal vein thrombosis several other pathologies have been proposed. Oedema of the bowel itself may cause pain and acute pancreatitis can occur secondary to the abnormalities in lipid metabolism associated with nephrotic syndrome. It has also been reported that low serum amino acid levels are associated with abdominal pain.

It is always worth considering carefully the indication for laparotomy in nephrotic syndrome since it is a potential hazard in such compromized subjects.

Case 19

Mrs R. G.

A 36-year-old female weaver presents to casualty with dyspnoea and oedema and gives the following history. At the age of 9 a tuberculous cervical lymph node was removed though no further treatment was given. At 18 years of age, following an episode of painless haematuria an intravenous urogram showed a small scarred left kidney with calcification and irregular cavitation. 'Acid-fast' bacilli bacilli were isolated in the urine and a course of streptomycin and para aminosalicylic acid (PAS) given for one year (although the patient later admitted poor compliance). Two years later following an episode of acute left-sided pyelonephritis an IVU showed a non functioning left kidney and a left nephrectomy was performed. Histologically the kidney contained acid fast bacilli (AFB) indicating that the disease was possibly still active so a further course of treatment was started. Later the same year frequency of micturition due to a fibrosed bladder was treated by colocystoplasty, in which a patch of colon is used to increase the size of the bladder.

She remained well until 7 years ago when she had a further episode of haematuria while living in Nigeria. She returned to England for tests. No AFB were isolated and further chemotherapy was withheld.

Her present complaint was of slowly progressive dyspnoea with orthopnoea and ankle oedema. On examination she was pale and tachypnoeic. Blood pressure was 230/130 mmHg, pulse 90 regular, JVP raised 4 cm and the apex was displaced to the left of the mid clavicular line with a triple cardiac rhythm. There was 5 cm hepatomegaly and a few crepitations at the lung bases. Fundi showed haemorrhages and exudates with arteriovenous nipping.

Urine contained blood + albumin + and blood results showed urea 27 mmol/ℓ (162 mg/100 ml), creatinine 780 μmol/ℓ (8.8 mg/100 ml), bicarbonate 9 mmol/ℓ, K 4.3 mmol/ℓ, Cl 114 mmolℓ, albumin 35 g/ℓ, Hb 8.1 g/dl, WCC 10.2 × 10^9/ℓ. Chest x-ray showed mild venous congestion.

Questions

1. What is the diagnosis?
2. What further tests would you like to perform?
3. What is the treatment?

Comment

The diagnosis is chronic renal failure with fluid overload and metabolic acidosis. In view of the history tuberculosis is the most likely cause. The further tests required are to exclude currently active disease and to see if there is any treatable obstructive element to the renal failure.

A chest x-ray should be performed and three early morning urines of sufficient volume (100 ml) sent for microscopy and incubation. A sterile pyuria need not indicate active disease in a previously treated patient. When the usual method of intravenous urography and retrograde pyelography prove unsatisfactory in defining the renal state, a CT body scan may be helpful in looking for enlarged intra-abdominal lymph nodes and in excluding ureteric obstruction. In view of the nature of the disease and the history with bladder involvement a micturating cystogram is useful in this case to define any ureteric reflux.

Renal tuberculosis accounts for 1% of patients with chronic renal failure in Europe reaching dialysis or transplantation. Renal TB usually occurs as a late complication of pulmonary disease, there being in severe cases massive caseous destruction and fibrosis within the renal parenchyma, obstructive uropathy caused by TB granulation or fibrosis within the pelvicalyceal systems, ureters or bladder. The presentations of genitourinary TB are those of obstructive uropathy, haematuria or chronic cystitis. Chronic renal insufficiency is rarely the first manifestation of renal tuberculosis.

If in doubt about the activity of the disease in a patient presenting with chronic renal failure treatment is essential as there is a high risk of reactivation of TB either because of uraemic immunosuppression or at transplantation because of the immunosuppressive drugs. Chemotherapy should be with triple therapy (isoniazid, ethambutol, rifampicin) for three months, continuing for a year on isoniazid and rifampicin. In uraemia dosages need to be reduced for ethambutol and isoniazid and blood levels need to be monitored.

A small point in this case is that the dyspnoea was aggrevated by the metabolic acidosis with a pH 7.18, base excess -17.5 mmol/ℓ, P_{CO_2} 20 mmHg and P_{O_2} 100 mmHg. This probably reflects tubular damage caused by the tuberculosis. This lady's remaining kidney was small with dilatation of the collecting system, pelvis and ureter but no evidence of obstruction. There was no evidence of active tuberculosis. The lesson from this case is that sub-optimal treatment (the patient admitted to missing her medication) and poor follow-up can lead to chronic renal failure which may be avoidable with adequate early treatment.

Case 20

Mr A. P.

A 50-year-old electrician was referred to surgical outpatients complaining of low back pain, following a fall 2 years previously. He had incidentally mentioned he had been passing 'frothy urine'. In the clinic an additional complaint of intermittent episodes of lower abdominal pain was noted but no other symptoms of renal or gastrointestinal disease were forthcoming.

Routine urinalysis demonstrated 300 mg% of albumin, blood pressure was 155/90 mmHg, there was no clinical abnormality of peripheral joints, straight leg raising was unimpaired and a full range of spinal movements was performed without pain or limitation. There was a scar posteriorly at the level of the left tenth rib, from a surgical drainage of an empyema at the age of 15 years. Initial investigations were reported as follows: ESR 38 mm/hour; spinal radiographs minor degenerative changes only; sacroiliac joints, normal; MSU no abnormalities; plasma albumin 29 gm/ℓ; plasma urea 4.7 mmol/ℓ (28 mg/100 ml). He was referred for a nephrological opinion, where a history of chronic cough, productive of purulent sputum was obtained. This had developed following an illness at the age of 12 years which the patient described as pneumonia. He had not smoked for 25 years. Physical signs on examination were bilateral basal crepitations and localized rhonchi at the left base. Investigations: Hb 16.8 g/dl; WCC, $10 \times 10^9/\ell$ with a normal differential; ESR 42 mm/hour; LE cells, not seen; ANF negative; plasma creatinine 100 µmol/ℓ (0.11 mg/100 ml); 24 hour urine protein 12 g; creatinine clearance 91 ml/minute; serum IgG 4.4 gm/ℓ; serum IgA 2.8 g/ℓ; serum IgM 1.1 g/ℓ; serum electrophoresis showed reduced levels of albumin and gamma globulins with an increase in alpha 2 globulins but with no monoclonal peak. Urine electrophoresis revealed gross generalized proteinuria only. Chest x-ray demonstrated basal fibrotic changes, pleural thickening and cystic bronchiectasis, some of the cystic areas having fluid levels.

Questions

1. List the major histopathological types and approximate incidence of adult patients in the UK with nephrotic syndrome (NS).
2. What is the diagnosis in this patient and how is it confirmed?

Comment

Between 5 and 10% of adults with NS, and having renal biopsies, in the UK ultimately prove to have amyloid disease. A further 5–10% have SLE or diabetes, 10% focal glomerulosclerosis and most of the rest, approximately 25% each, have minimal change, membranous and proliferative histology.

Ancillary investigations such as rectal or gingival biopsies may reveal amyloid deposits, but the tentative diagnosis, as in this patient, requires confirmation with renal biopsy and appropriate staining with Congo red, which, under polarized light gives a green/yellow dichromic birefringence.

Amyloid, an insoluble protein, which is usually but not invariably deposited in the glomeruli, occasionally fails to take up the dye, in which case it can be differentiated from diabetic glomerulosclerosis by its characteristic fibrillary structure, visible on electron microscopy. Initially the deposits are mesangial and subendothelial in position and may extend through the basement membrane obliterating the vascular lumina. On light microscopy it can resemble membranous nephropathy unless the section is specifically stained for amyloid.

Much of the confusion about amyloidosis stems from the classification as 'primary' or 'secondary' in respect of apparent underlying cause and the pattern of tissues involved. Different types of amyloid are composed of approximately 95% fibrils and 5% amyloid P component, the latter being a constant feature which is antigenically identical with a serum glycoprotein, serum amyloid P component (SAP).

It has recently been reported that distinctive SAP deposition (demonstrated by immunofluorescent anti-SAP) occurs in various types of primary and secondary glomerulonephritis. The fibrillary component of amyloid may be of two types; in 'primary' and 'myeloma associated' amyloidosis it appears to be composed predominantly of Lambda light chains (AL) whereas that of familial Mediterranean fever and following chronic inflammatory diseases such as osteomyelitis, tuberculosis, bronchiectasis, Crohn's disease, ulcerative colitis, rheumatoid arthritis and ankylosing spondylitis as well as that associated with malignancy (Hodgkin's disease, carcinoma and even hypernephroma) is antigenically distinct, and designated amyloid A (AA) protein. Normal serum also contains amounts of AA (SAA), the level of which increases with age.

Patients with 'secondary' amyloidosis usually present with nephrotic syndrome. Casts and microscopic haematuria may or may not be present. This patient illustrates the well-recognized phenomenon of a delay of many years from the onset of the underlying disease (bronchiectasis) to the development of clinically recognizable renal malfunction. The extensive nature of the bronchiectatic changes precluded surgical resection in this man and he was advised to perform postural drainage daily, and was put on long-term antibiotics. Effective treatment of the primary insult may arrest or even reverse the course of renal involvement.

Currently, three years from the original presentation, he is needing therapy for hypertension, renal function is unimpaired and he continues with prophylactic antibiotics. The proteinuria is stable. His abdominal pain was attributed to extensive colonic diverticulitis.

Case 21

Mr P. B.

An 18-year-old cost clerk was admitted to casualty as an emergency following a grand mal fit. He was unable to give a history but his parents explained that he had been well until two weeks previously when he developed a sore throat, which was successfully treated with antibiotics. His urine had become a rusty brown colour with decreasing volumes over the previous three to four days and he had been complaining of headaches, feeling generally tired with episodes of nausea. On the day of admission he had slept most of the time and had two grand mal fits before being brought to hospital. There was no family history of renal disease or epilepsy. On examination he was drowsy, disorientated and uncooperative. He had a petechial rash on his arms and legs with bruising on his thighs. Temperature was 37.2 °C. Blood pressure was initially 130/80 mmHg rising to 180/130 mmHg within one hour. Pulse 90 regular, the apex beat was not displaced and the heart sounds normal with no murmurs. There was no oedema and the chest was clear. His throat was injected. Neurological examination showed good power in all limbs but with increased tone. Reflexes were brisk and the plantar responses both flexor. There was no neck stiffness. Fundi showed bilateral papilloedema with haemorrhages.

He was given intravenous diazoxide to control his blood pressure and transferred to the ward. Urgent results showed urea 47 mmol/ℓ

(282 mg/100 ml), K 5.7 mmol/ℓ, creatinine 1800 μmol/ℓ (20.4 mg/100 ml), Hb 9.9 g/dl, WCC 4.6 × 10^9/ℓ, retics 5%, platelets 60 × 10^9/ℓ. The blood film showed microangiopathy with target cells and schistocytes. FDPs 1:128 (normal 1:8). Prothrombin time 19 seconds (control 15 seconds). Thrombin time 45 seconds (control 36 seconds). Coombs' test negative. ECG showed a normal axis and sinus rhythm. Chest x-ray was normal with no cardiomegaly. Abdominal x-ray showed normal sized kidneys.

Questions

1. What is the diagnosis?
2. What is the treatment?
3. What would the biopsy show?

Comment

This is a case of acute renal failure following a sore throat, which could be due to a post streptococcal glomerulonephritis but there is a further factor to take into account. The characteristic blood film showing fragmented and distorted red cells with reticulocytosis make the diagnosis haemolytic uraemic syndrome (HUS). This is a rare disease which occurs most frequently in young children under the age of 4 years, but is being increasingly recognized in young adults, and especially following pregnancy. An infective factor either viral or bacterial is thought to be the 'trigger' though no one organism has been implicated. In children the disease is often less severe than the adults with 90% survival though some may progress to chronic renal failure. In adults acute deaths are often due to neurological involvement. Malignant hypertension often occurs and may reflect acute renal damage or be a primary event. In this case there is no evidence of long standing hypertension as both the ECG and chest x-ray were normal.

Pathologically HUS is due to a thrombosis within small arterioles and capillaries mainly in the kidneys but it can affect other organs such as the brain giving rise to neurological signs in the absence of severe hypertension. When the haemolytic blood picture is associated with neurological features with little evidence of renal involvement the diagnostic label of thrombotic thrombocytopaenic purpura (TTP) is used. These two syndromes may well represent two ends of a spectrum with similar pathological processes involving different organs dependent upon the triggering mechanism.

Recent workers have proposed that in some patients the syndrome may be due to an inherited deficiency of prostacyclin production by vessel walls. With a suitable trigger mechanism this results in increased platelet stickiness to the vessel wall and thrombosis. This may only be important in some cases though treatment with infused prostacyclin has been successful occasionally. Other treatments which have had some success are infusion of fresh frozen plasma, plasmaphoresis, and whole blood exchange. The treatments are aimed at either replacing a missing factor (e.g. prostacyclin) or removing a trigger factor. Theoretically if the deposition of fibrin is part of the sequence of events the use of heparin would be expected to be beneficial, though as yet this has not been shown in adults.

A renal biopsy is not diagnostic of HUS but is necessary to exclude glomerulonephritis. Characteristically it should show thrombosis within small arterioles and capillaries with little glomerular damage. In this patient the biopsy showed minor changes in the glomeruli, wrinkling of the basement membrane indicative of ischaemia, and fibrin deposits within capillary loops and arterioles. Despite heparin and plasmaphoresis renal function did not recover and chronic haemodialysis was commenced. Blood pressure control remained a problem eventually requiring a nephrectomy.

Case 22

Mr J. S.

A previously fit 50-year-old cost clerk had complained for a year of intermittent left loin pain. An IVU showed radioopaque calculi in the pelvis of the left kidney. He had never passed stones and there was no family history of calculi. His renal function was normal with a urea 5.2 mmol/ℓ (31 mg/100 ml) and creatinine 65 μmol/ℓ (0.73 mg/100 ml). A left pyelolithotomy was performed. Four hours post operatively he was oozing blood from the incision, though his blood pressure was 140/80. A single unit of packed cells was ordered. While this transfusion was in progress signs of circulatory collapse occurred, with a blood pressure 60/20, temperature 40 °C and rigors. Three litres of dextrose and saline were given with an improvement in the blood pressure though he became oliguric and failed to respond to 1 g of intravenous frusemide. Eighteen hours after the operation he was transferred for management of acute renal failure. On examination he was an obese man who was tachypnoeic. Pulse was 100 regular and blood pressure 140/80, JVP raised 4 cm and his heart had a triple rhythm. There was ankle oedema, 2 cm hepatomegaly and basal crepitations. The urine was a rusty brown colour and positive for blood and protein on dipstick testing. Results showed Na 128 mmol/ℓ, K 4.7 mmol/ℓ, urea 14.4 mmol/ℓ (86 mg/100 ml), creatinine 300 μmol/ℓ (3.4 mg/100 ml), Hb 13.1 g/dl, WCC 16.4 × 10^9/ℓ, platelets 93 × 10^9/ℓ with a microangiopathic picture. PCV 37.5%. Bilirubin 52 μmol/ℓ (2.6 mg/100 ml), prothrombin time 24 seconds (control 15 seconds), Kaolin cephalin time 38 seconds (control 38 seconds). Thrombin time 33 seconds (control 29 seconds). FDPs 1:128 (normal 1:8). Blood cultures were sterile. Chest x-ray showed pulmonary congestion with small bilateral effusions.

Questions

1. What is the diagnosis?
2. What is the treatment?

Comment

This episode of acute renal failure was associated with hypotension, rigors, and disseminated intravascular coagulation. The three most likely causes are acute blood loss, septicaemia or incompatible blood transfusion. Acute blood loss would give hypotension but not the rigors. Septicaemia fits the hypotension, rigors and disseminated intravascular coagulation. However sepsis rarely occurs within hours of the initial event as in this case, time being necessary for the bacteria to multiply and produce sufficient endotoxin. The third possibility of an incompatible blood transfusion is most likely. The hypotension and rigors occurred whilst the blood was being given and a raised bilirubin is indicative of haemolysis.

On further investigation the patient was blood group O and the pack of transfused cells was group A (a mistake having been made by the nursing staff in giving the wrong pack). Two patients with the same name had had blood crossmatched that day and the hospital numbers had not been checked against the numbers on the blood packs. Group O patients possess cytotoxic anti-A and anti-B antibody, therefore the transfused A cells were haemolysed by the patient's anti-A.

Further laboratory investigations to support this are the frank red colour of the serum indicating free haemoglobin which has leaked from the haemolysed red cells. The urine was rusty brown and on stick testing was strongly positive for blood (which tests for the haem moiety) but only a few red cells were present on microscopy indicative of haemoglobinuria rather than haematuria.

The exact cause of the renal damage in haemolysis is debated. Both disseminated intravascular coagulation and haemoglobin cast formation have been implicated.

The basis of treatment is to stop the causative transfusion and restore effective blood volume. Exchange transfusions may be indicated at an early stage in severe cases and the urine output should be maintained. Not all incompatible blood transfusions cause haemolysis severe enough to produce acute renal failure or even a fall in haemoglobin. Other causes of haemolysis and renal failure are the autoimmune haemolytic anaemias, glucose-6-phosphate dehydrogenase deficiency, sickle cell crisis, and the induction of abortion by interuterine hypertonic solutions.

In this case the disseminated intravascular coagulation and evidence of haemolysis settled within two days, however the urea and creatinine rose. Peritoneal dialysis was performed for 6 days before the patient's renal function improved. Three weeks following the episode his urea and creatinine were normal and further recovery was uneventful.

Case 23

Mr J. G.

In the course of a medical examination for insurance purposes, a 36-year-old policeman was found on dipstick testing to have albumin but no sugar or blood in the urine. There was no history indicative of antecedent nephritis, urinary tract infection or obstructive uropathy, and no suggestion of analgesic abuse, systemic disorder or familial renal disease. He had never been aware of ankle swelling or haematuria, and there were no abnormalities to find on clinical examination, specifically he was normotensive without oedema or palpable kidneys.

Repeated urinalyses confirmed the presence of persisting but asymptomatic proteinuria both in early morning urine samples and specimens obtained when ambulant. Detailed investigations revealed normal haematological indices, normal renal function, a plasma albumin of 47 gm/ℓ but proteinuria of between 2 and 6 g per day. Serological tests for connective tissue disease were all negative, as was the WR, and no paraprotein was detected on electrophoresis of serum or concentrated urine. Similarly, there was no abnormality on microscopy or culture of urine, an IVU was also normal and plasma urate was within the normal range. Renal biopsy was performed.

In the following 3 years the proteinuria slowly diminished in quantity to within normal limits and his renal function remained unaffected. However, in the subsequent 7 years his blood pressure rose to a level requiring treatment with a thiazide diuretic. He continues in remission with normal renal function and has remained completely asymptomatic throughout.

Questions

1. What are the currently accepted indications for performing a renal biopsy?
2. What is the significance of glomerular disease presenting as asymptomatic proteinuria rather than a nephrotic syndrome?

Comment

Although the indications for attempting a percutaneous renal biopsy have varied over the years since its introduction, there is now general agreement that it may, with certain provisions, be desirable in any of the following circumstances: 24 hour urine protein in excess of 1 g; unexplained haematuria, once lower tract disease and other identifiable renal causes e.g. tumour or calculi are excluded; unexplained renal failure and, to determine the cause of abnormal function in a transplanted kidney e.g. ATN, rejection and recurrence of the primary disease.

Examination of the tissue obtained by light and electron microscopy, and by immunofluorescent techniques has allowed the development of a sophisticated classification of glomerular disease which may be of assistance in assessing prognosis and likely response to treatment, e.g. in minimal change disease.

Proteinuria can be due to:

(a) prerenal causes such as myeloma, where light chains may appear in the urine (Bence–Jones proteinuria),

(b)   glomerular disorders including the immune complex mediated diseases and infiltrative lesions such as amyloid as well as orthostatic, exercise induced and febrile proteinuria,

(c)   tubular disease, and

(d)   infection anywhere in the renal tract.

It can occur also in toxaemia of pregnancy.

The term asymptomatic proteinuria is used to imply glomerular proteinuria which is insufficient to cause development of a nephrotic syndrome. Analysis of a variety of series of patients with glomerular disease nearly always demonstrates a better prognosis, as judged by survival curves, if presenting with asymptomatic proteinuria rather than a nephrotic syndrome. An exception to the rule has recently been suggested in patients with SLE.

This patient proved to have a mesangial proliferative glomerulonephritis with an increase in both mesangial cells and matrix in all glomeruli examined, but no endocapillary proliferation or basement membrane abnormalities. Immunofluorescent studies were unavailable. Mesangioproliferative disease may present in a variety of ways, as a nephrotic syndrome and not uncommonly with asymptomatic proteinuria, and both macroscopic and microscopic haematuria are well-recognized manifestations with or without accompanying proteinuria. Usually there is no concurrent or antecedent associated illness but it may sometimes appear to represent the healing phase of acute post infectious glomerulonephritis or be associated with SLE or Henoch–Schönlein purpura. The majority of patients have an excellent prognosis with no sequelae, particularly those presenting with asymptomatic proteinuria. Some studies have documented a response in the proteinuria following steroid therapy but there may be difficulty in differentiating this condition from minimal change disease, particularly in the absence of immunofluorescent data. Similarly, subsequent biopsies very occasionally result in reclassification on a pathological basis into focal glomerulosclerosis or mesangiocapillary disease.

Case 24

Mrs D. B.

A 27-year-old housewife was admitted to the local maternity hospital, 22 weeks into her first pregnancy, with a 48 hour history of blood loss per vaginum. Her previous medical history was unremarkable and the pregnancy had otherwise been proceeding normally. On admission, the uterine size was consistent with dates, blood pressure was 110/60 mmHg, there was no oedema and urinalysis was negative for protein. The vaginal blood loss continued, accompanied by clear amniotic fluid. After one week ultrasonic scan failed to demonstrate the presence of any amniotic fluid, confirming the diagnosis of premature rupture of the membranes. The combination of undetectable fetal heart sounds and a persisting pyrexia led to the decision to complete the missed abortion.

Over the next 40 hours the patient received 5 ℓ of intravenous fluids containing oxytocin in the recommended doses (2–5 milli-units/minute) but a vaginal delivery did not ensue. She gradually became drowsy and disorientated and eventually had a grand-mal convulsion of a few minutes duration. In the immediate postictal phase blood pressure was 120/70 mmHg and blood sugar 6 mmol/ℓ.

Questions

1. What single biochemical result confirmed the clinical diagnosis?
2. What is the physiological explanation?

Comment

The intravenous fluid used for the infusion had been 5% dextrose and examination of balance charts revealed a total urine output of less than 500 ml in the 36 hours prior to the convulsion. Plasma sodium postictally was 114 mmol/ℓ and potassium 3 mmol/ℓ. Further investigations revealed a serum osmolality of 230 mmol/kg (normal range 275–295) and an inappropriately high urine osmolality of 296 mmol/kg.

This patient had suffered from the convulsions associated with water intoxication. The results indicated an inappropriate, in this case iatrogenic, antidiuretic hormone-like syndrome. Oxytocin has

ADH action and prolonged administration with only dextrose solution led to marked water retention.

The immediate management was with intravenous frusemide and phenytoin and a small slow infusion of hypertonic saline, calculated to bring the plasma sodium to just greater than 120 mmol/ℓ. In a less dramatic situation, simple water restriction would be sufficient. Rapid fluid shifts from water-logged cells by administration of larger volumes of hypertonic fluids are best avoided. The abortion was completed using a prostaglandin preparation.

She remained comatose for 14 hours and continued to have focal fits for 6 days. Full subjective and objective neurological recovery took many weeks.

In virtually identical circumstances a fatal outcome has been reported. Oxytocin is also reported to cause hypertension, subarachnoid haemorrhage and cardiac arrhythmias as well as other complications to the pregnancy such as uterine rupture.

Other causes of hyponatraemia
1. Gastrointestinal losses of solute without adequate replacement, e.g. vomiting, diarrhoea.
2. Inappropriate secretion of ADH with
    (a) malignancy; especially oat cell carcinoma of lung but also pancreatic carcinoma
    (b) central nervous system pathology; brain tumour and encephalitis
    (c) drugs; such as chlorpropamide and vincristine
    (d) pulmonary pathology; TB and pneumonia
3. Addison's disease
4. Congestive cardiac failure, especially in conjunction with diuretic therapy.
5. Hepatic cirrhosis
6. Renal disease
    (a) acute renal failure
    (b) salt losing nephritis
7. Psychogenic polydipsia
8. Pseudohyponatraemia
    (a) paraproteinaemia
    (b) hyperlipidaemia

Case 25

Mrs F. H.

A 74-year-old housewife was referred to the orthopaedic department because of progressive back pain, which was worse on bend-
ing and made dressing difficult. X-rays of the spine and pelvis
showed the features of osteomalacia with reduced bone density,
biconcavity of the vertebral bodies and pseudofractures (Looser's
zones) in the pelvis and femora. Urine testing with dipsticks was
positive for glucose and protein. She was therefore referred for a
medical opinion with a diagnosis of osteomalacia and possibly
diabetes mellitus. There was no previous or family history of renal
disease and apart from the back pain she had been quite well
except for a myocardial infarction six years previously. On examination she was slightly obese with localized rib tenderness. Blood
pressure was 190/90 mmHg and the pulse 90 regular and with no
oedema. Urine testing showed 2% glycosuria with Clinitest and a
concomitant blood sugar of 4.2 mmol/ℓ (76 mg/100 ml). Other
results were Na 139 mmol/ℓ, K 3.0 mmol/ℓ, Cl 113 mmol/ℓ, urea 6.6
mmol/ℓ (40 mg/100 ml), creatinine 110 μmol/ℓ (1.3 mg/100 ml),
calcium 2.3 mmol/ℓ (9.4 mg/100 ml), PO_4 0.54 mmol/ℓ (1.73 mg/100
ml), alkaline phosphatase 122 IU/ℓ, total protein 90 g/ℓ, albumin 39
g/ℓ, urate 0.14 mmol/ℓ (2.3 mg/100 ml), Hb 12.5 g/dl, WCC 9.2 ×
10^9/ℓ with a normal differential, platelets 200 × 10^9/ℓ, ESR 50 mm/
hour. A capillary astrup showed pH 7.31, PCO$_2$ 33.5 mmHg, PO$_2$ 70
mmHg, base excess −9.5, actual bicarbonate 15.5 mmol/ℓ, standard
bicarbonate 17 mmol/ℓ with a urine pH 6.6. Creatinine clearance
was 50 ml/minute with 2 g proteinuria per day. There was gross
generalized aminoaciduria on chromatography. Urine osmolality
after an overnight water deprivation test was 550 mmol/kg. A bone
biopsy confirmed the diagnosis of osteomalacia.

Questions

1. What is the diagnosis?
2. What further tests would you like to do?
3. What is the treatment?

Comment

The positive findings in this lady are first osteomalacia (confirmed by bone biopsy and indicated by radiology, low phosphate and raised alkaline phosphatase), and secondly evidence of gross tubular dysfunction. A proximal tubular abnormality is illustrated by renal glycosuria (2% glycosuria with a normal blood sugar) and generalized aminoaciduria. The distal tubules show lack of concentrating ability after water deprivation (osmolality 550 mmol/kg, normal 700–900 mmol/kg) and an acidification defect (a systemic acidosis with pH 7.31 and a urine pH of only 6.6). There is also hypokalaemia and hyperchloraemia indicative of distal tubular dysfunction. Although not diagnostic the hypophosphataemia and hypouricaemia are probably due to high phosphate and urate clearances. The osteomalacia is therefore secondary to the tubular defects and is the presenting feature of this adult Fanconi's syndrome.

This has not completely solved the problem for in idiopathic adult Fanconi's syndrome with distal and proximal tubular damage the usual presentation is in early middle age with bone pain. It is a rare disease which may be of recessive or dominant inheritance. The acquired, more common form of the disease, secondary to a paraprotein is therefore more likely. Evidence for this is supported by the raised ESR and total protein. Fanconi's syndrome can occur with either a benign paraprotein or myeloma. Further tests should therefore include a bone marrow, skeletal survey and immunoelectrophoresis of serum and urine. In this case there were 20% atypical plasma cells, no lytic bone lesions but an IgG Kappa paraprotein was found in the serum with free Kappa light chains in the urine (Bence-Jones proteinuria).

Another form of Fanconi syndrome presents in childhood and is due to an autosomal recessive gene. Cystinosis, in which deposits of cystine occur in many organs also produces this tubular syndrome. Crystals can be seen in the conjunctivae, cornea and bone marrow.

The prognosis in the childhood form is poor but that of the adult idiopathic variety is good. In the secondary type the prognosis is related to that of the underlying disorder. Treatment consists of correcting the hypokalaemic acidosis with sodium bicarbonate and potassium citrate (Scholl's solution). Osteomalacia is treated with vitamin D and the paraprotein is treated with cytotoxic therapy such as melphalan and prednisolone or cyclophosphamide. In this patient her myeloma progressed and the patient died of bronchopneumonia although her osteomalacia had been cured.

Case 26

Miss P. C.

A 23-year-old single unemployed insulin dependent (Type I) diabetic girl was referred to the renal clinic for management of her renal failure. Diabetes was diagnosed at the age of 3 years when she presented with weight loss, polyuria and polydipsia. Since then her diabetes had been well controlled with a variety of regimens, but most recently taking twice daily soluble insulin. Over the previous year she has had several hypoglycaemic attacks even though her urine has been showing 0.5–1% glycosuria. She has had difficulty with her eyesight and has received laser photocoagulation for proliferative retinopathy. Proteinuria was first detected on clinic visits at the age of 20. This was intermittent at first with months of negative results, though it has been consistently positive for the past 2 years.

One year ago she had an episode of severe colicky left loin pain followed two days later by the passing of a piece of 'white matter' in her urine.

On examination she was a pleasant normally developed girl. There was bilateral ankle oedema but no evidence of heart failure. Lying pulse was 90 beats per minute, blood pressure 130/80 mmHg, standing pulse 90 beats per minute, blood pressure 100/60 mmHg. Fundi showed proliferative retinopathy with scarring of photocoagulation. Ankle jerks were absent.

Results showed urea 21 mmol/ℓ (126 mg/100 ml), creatinine 625 μmol/ℓ (7.1 mg/100 ml). Blood sugar 6.8 mmol/ℓ (122 mg/100 ml). Urine 1% glycosuria. A 24 hour urine contained 1 g of unselective proteinuria.

Questions

1. What is the prognosis?
2. What is the cause of the oedema?
3. What treatment is available?
4. What was the cause of the loin pain?

Comment

This young girl fits the typical profile of a patient with end stage progressive diabetic nephropathy. Although she is young at presentation she has already had diabetes for 17 years. Older patients with diabetes are more likely to die from ischaemic heart disease before diabetic nephropathy has advanced. Diabetic nephropathy nearly always develops in association with other complications unlike retinopathy and neuropathy which can occur alone.

Proteinuria on dipstick testing is usually the first sign of the disease though histological changes without proteinuria can occur much earlier. A positive dipstick occurs in up to 15% of diabetics but renal impairment hardly ever occurs without proteinuria. Proteinuria is usually less than 1 g/day for the nephrotic syndrome only occurs in advanced disease, prior to terminal renal failure. The time interval between the discovery of proteinuria and deterioration of renal function varies greatly and may be up to 18 years. Once however the blood urea is raised the disease often progresses rapidly to terminal renal failure within two years. Oedema may occur before the serum albumin falls or the blood urea rises and is possibly associated with neuropathy. Neuropathy, sensory, motor or autonomic is a nearly universal associated finding with diabetic nephropathy but may be accentuated by the uraemia. Autonomic neuropathy may produce a neurogenic bladder with the serious problem of urinary tract infection and is a relative contraindication to renal transplantation. Postural hypotension is another complication caused by autonomic neuropathy and causes difficulties with fluid balance and blood pressure control. Arterial atheroma is common in diabetic subjects and if renal replacement therapy is commenced, myocardial infarction is the most frequent cause of death.

Histologically the diabetic kidney is characterized by thickening of the glomerular basement membrane and capillary walls with mesangial cell proliferation. This produces as a rare feature nodular lesions within the glomerulus (the Kimmelstiel–Wilson kidney).

Once renal failure is established urine glucose measurements can be misleading. The requirement for insulin may also decrease because of a reduced catabolism of insulin by the diseased kidney. The loin pain was caused by the shedding of a necrotic renal papilla. This occurs because of thrombosis of small blood vessels in the kidney as part of the generalized arterial disease.

Treatment is aimed at obtaining very good control of the diabetes with regular blood sugar tests. Dialysis is best started early in these patients. If there is autonomic neuropathy, haemodialysis may be difficult because of the brittle fluid balance control, and retinopathy increases the potential risk of intraocular haemorrhage due to heparinization for dialysis. CAPD has become popular for treating diabetic renal failure, administering insulin intraperitoneally with the dialysis fluid. However with deteriorating eyesight this may become a difficult mode of treatment for the patient to manage alone.

Transplantation is possible though the results are much worse than in age matched non-diabetic patients.

The patient described was started on CAPD which she performed very successfully without peritonitis until she received a successful cadaver renal transplant.

Case 27

Mrs J. S.

A 63-year-old female dress shop assistant had hypertension for 15 years. Eight years ago she was investigated when chest x-ray, ECG, intravenous urogram, MSU, urea and electrolytes, thyroid function, uric acid, haemoglobin white cell count and ESR were all normal. She was treated with methyldopa and propranolol but became depressed and agitated. The methyldopa was changed to debrisoquine with symptomatic improvement in her mood though poor blood pressure control. Bendrofluazide (5 mg) was added 5 years ago and the debrisoquine changed to hydralazine 50 mg tds 3 years ago.

She presented as an urgency 6 months ago to the rheumatology department with throbbing and swelling of the lateral aspect of the right ankle which was hot, reddened and tender. Serum urate was 0.4 mmol/ℓ (6.6 mg/100 ml) and 24 hour urinary urate 2.3 mmol/ℓ (38 mg/100 ml). X-rays showed no abnormality and joint aspiration was unsuccessful. Clinically she was thought to have gout so the bendrofluazide was stopped. Her blood pressure rose and the hydralazine was increased to 50 mg qds. On discharge: Hb 10.0 g/dl, WCC 4.1 $\times$ 10^9/ℓ (lymphocytes 19%), urea 13.7 mmol/ℓ (84 mg/100 ml), creatinine 160 μmol/ℓ (1.8 mg/100 ml), ANF positive, anti-DNA antibodies 22 units/ml. At follow-up in clinic she was complaining of tiredness, nausea and dizziness with ankle swelling. She was admitted as an urgency and on examination blood pressure was 220/110 mmHg. JVP raised 4 cm with a triple rhythm and an apical systolic murmur. There were basal crepitations and 1 cm hepatomegaly and a palpable spleen. Fundi showed arteriovenous nipping. Results: urea 23.5 mmol/ℓ (141 mg/100 ml), creatinine 340 μmol/ℓ (3.85 mg/100 ml), albumin 34 g/ℓ, Hb 7.1 g/dl, WCC 4.2 × $10^9/\ell$ (85% neutrophils, 9% lymphocytes), platelets 253 × $10^9/\ell$, ESR 91 mm/hour, retics 1.1%, 24 hour urine protein 1.6 g/24 hour, ANF positive, anti-DNA antibodies 42 units/ml. Clotting studies revealed prolongation of prothrombin time (PT) and thrombin time (TT). Fibrinogen normal, serum FDPs normal. There was a circulating inhibitor to coagulation. Direct Coombs' test negative.

Questions

1. What is the diagnosis?
2. What is the treatment?
3. What is the prognosis?

Comment

The diagnosis is hydralazine induced systemic lupus erythematosus (SLE). On stopping the hydralazine there was no further deterioration in the haematological and biochemical tests — but no improvement. Prednisolone was therefore started, initially at 100 mg a day reducing by 10 mg a week and changing to an alternate day schedule. Three months later: Hb 11.9 g/dl, WCC 6.7 × $10^9/\ell$ (64% neutrophils, 18% lymphocytes), ESR 32 mm/hour, urea 13.8 mmol/ℓ (83 mg/100 ml), creatinine 110 μmol/ℓ (1.2 mg/100 ml). Coagulation was still abnormal with KCT 72 seconds (control 34.5 seconds).

Drug induced SLE is thought to occur in two patterns, an 'allergic' type due to such drugs as penicillin, tetracycline, streptomycin, reserpine, methyl dopa, phenylbutazone, chlorthalidone and griseofulvin, which is usually seen soon after starting the drug and is not dose related. There is a high correlation between a positive antinuclear factor and clinical symptoms.

The second pattern to which hydralazine, isoniazid, procaineamide, chlorpromazine, phenytoin, primidone and ethosuximide conform is thought to be dose related. Up to 40% of patients taking these drugs develop a positive antinuclear factor; but less than 10% develop the clinical symptoms of SLE.

Clinically the symptoms of drug induced SLE are indistinguishable from the idiopathic disease though renal involvement is less common. Serologically the antinuclear factor is positive though DNA binding (antibodies to native double stranded DNA), is lower in drug induced lupus. Hydralazine induced lupus is a disease of women of tissue type HLA DR 4 and with slow acetylator status. Hydralazine is normally metabolized by acetylation in the liver. There is a bimodal population distribution of the activity of this enzymic step (fast and slow acetylators). Slow acetylators cannot metabolize hydralazine as quickly and therefore higher serum levels result.

The treatment is to discontinue the offending drug, though this does not always bring about reversal of the disease. If symptoms persist the treatment should be that of conventional lupus. Because of the risk of hydralazine induced systemic lupus the dosage should not exceed 150 mg/day, especially in females.

Case 28

Mr P. W.

A 28-year-old sales representative gave a history of macroscopic haematuria on three separate occasions in the preceding year, which he associated with a sore throat and 'tonsillitis'. The episode which precipitated his admission followed an influenzal type illness with headache, sore throat and myalgia. The urine was uniformly blood stained. The history was otherwise unremarkable, specifically he had not had any symptoms suggestive of renal or urinary tract disease previously, nor was there any relevant family history. There were no abnormal findings on examination.

Urinalysis demonstrated numerous RBC but no proteinuria or casts. An IVU and cystoscopy at his local hospital revealed no abnormality, but microscopic haematuria persisted and he was referred for a nephrological opinion.

At this time he was normotensive with no significant proteinuria and normal renal function. The results of some other investigations were: ASOT raised at 600 Todd units, ESR 33 mm/hour, Hb 12 g/dl and MSU sterile. The only other detectable biochemical abnormality was a raised serum IgA level at 5.8 gm/ℓ (normal 1–4.25 g/ℓ) with normal urine and serum protein electrophoretic patterns. Serological investigations revealed the presence of persisting HBsAg along with HBcAb and HBeAb but with normal liver function tests.

Questions

1. What investigations are indicated?
2. What is the most likely diagnosis?

Comment

Haematuria has a variety of causes, however, in the absence of any family history (Alport's nephritis or benign familial haematuria) and in the presence of a normal IVU and cystoscopy, Berger's disease is a distinct possibility. This eponymous title refers to the combination of recurrent haematuria in association with a mesangial proliferative glomerulonephritis, where IgA is the predominant localizing immunoglobulin. Renal biopsy in this patient confirmed the diagnosis, with IgA distributed in a diffuse global and granular fashion predominantly in the mesangium.

This condition frequently has a benign course, but renal failure can ensue, and the same histopathology may recur in a transplanted kidney. An association between Berger's disease and HLA DRW4 has been reported, as has the observation of raised circulating IgA levels, although neither are essential for the diagnosis.

Five years since the onset of his haematuria he remains well with normal renal function and blood pressure, intermittent microscopic haematuria and an occasional 24 hour urine protein of more than 1 g. The significance of persisting hepatitis B surface antigenaemia is uncertain and does not appear to have been described as a feature of Berger's disease.

Other patients with the same diagnosis present with micro or macroscopic haematuria, with or without significant proteinuria. In some patients proteinuria may develop years after the original episode of haematuria. It is common for patients to report episodes of macroscopic haematuria following simple upper respiratory tract infections; intermittent microscopic haematuria frequently occurs in the absence of overt infection.

Causes of haematuria
It is important to remember that

(a) Tumour
(b) Trauma

(c) Pyogenic infection, and
(d) Calculi, at any site in the renal and urinary systems may be responsible.

Next consider

1. Systemic causes such as
    (a) anticoagulation
    (b) haemophilia
    (c) thrombocytopenia
    (d) hypertension
    (e) sickle cell disease
2. Intrinsic renal causes
    (a) glomerulonephritis
    (b) tuberculosis
    (c) polycystic disease
    (d) analgesic nephropathy
    (e) loin pain haematuria syndrome
3. Lower renal tract lesions
    (a) haemorrhagic cystitis (cyclophosphamide)
    (b) bilharzia
    (c) prostatitis
    (d) prostatic varices
    (e) urethral foreign bodies

Case 29

Mr J. H.

A 31-year-old male mechanical engineer was found to have a plasma potassium of 2.3 mmol/ℓ following appendicectomy. Post-operative recovery was rapid and uneventful, but hypokalaemia persisted despite oral and intravenous potassium chloride.

His only complaint was of occasional pins and needles in his fingers. He did not complain of weakness and considered his urine volume normal. He was subsequently admitted to a metabolic ward for investigation. After 12 days on a rigorous diet containing sodium 200 mmol/day and potassium 200 mmol/day, he remained well; blood pressure was 110/70 mmHg both lying and standing and urine volume averaged 2.5 ℓ/day. Investigations included plasma K 2.4

mmol/ℓ, plasma Na 136 mmol/ℓ, plasma Cl 85 mmol/ℓ, plasma bicarbonate 28 mmol/ℓ, arterial pH 7.43, base excess + 6.5, urine Na 190 mmol/day, urine K 185 mmol/day, faecal potassium 10 mmol/day, a normal IVP, plasma renin activity at 27 ng/ml/hour (expected less than 8 ng/ml/hour), and normal plasma aldosterone at 380 pmol/ℓ (normal 100–500 pmol/ℓ). Dietary sodium was then reduced to 20 mmol/day for 8 days with dietary potassium unchanged. At the end of this period body weight had fallen 2 kg, plasma sodium was 135 mmol/ℓ, plasma K 2.1 mmol/ℓ, plasma bicarbonate 27.5 mmol/ℓ, arterial pH 7.46, base excess + 4.5. Urine Na decreased to 18 mmol/day after 6 days and urine potassium remained equal to intake levels at 180–190 mmol/day. Plasma renin activity increased slightly to 45 ng/ml/hour and aldosterone to 500 pmol/ℓ.

Questions

1. What is the diagnosis?
2. What are postulated mechanisms of its pathogenesis?
3. How do you treat this patient?

Comment

Most of the body potassium (approx. 3500 mmol, 31–57 mmol/kg) is intracellular and the plasma level is a poor guide to the total stores. Although the deficit in this patient is likely to be large, its magnitude cannot be determined from the data.

Effects of potassium depletion on renal function include a vasopressin-resistant concentrating defect, increased secretion of renin by juxtaglomerular cells and of prostaglandin E by medullary interstitial cells and an increased urinary excretion of ammonium. Renal biopsy may show vacuolation of tubular cells and it is possible that interstitial nephritis can develop, although firm evidence for the latter in man is lacking. Clinically overt polyuria and myopathy may not be present unless the potassium deficit is large, and the lack of symptoms in this patient is not unusual.

The causes of renal potassium wasting may be classified according to the level of blood pressure and by acid-base state (*Table 29.1*). This patient is alkalotic and has a low blood pressure.

Surreptitious diuretic use may be suggested by an abnormal personality, but is often very difficult to establish. Diuretics may be detected in the blood or urine, but are present only intermittently and it is rarely possible to screen for all possibilities. The diagnosis

Table 29.1   Causes of excessive urinary potassium loss

High Blood Pressure	Normal or Low Blood Pressure

Mineralocorticoid excess:
  Conn's Syndrome
  Cushing's Syndrome
Overproduction of renin:
  Accelerated Hypertension
  Renal Artery Stenosis
  Renin Secreting Tumour
 	
Liddle's Syndrome
Liquorice Ingestion
	Systemic Acidosis
	  Renal Tubular Acidosis
	
	Systemic Alkalosis (or normal blood pH)
	  Diuretic Use
	  Metabolic Alkalosis
	  Bartter's Syndrome
	  Magnesium Deficiency

may be suggested by abnormal diurnal or day-to-day variation in urine volume and electrolyte content. There is often associated self-induced vomiting or laxative abuse. A search of the patient's belongings or questioning of relatives and the general practitioner may reveal the source of diuretics. In this patient, a stable personality, an orderly metabolic balance study and the incidental presentation make diuretic abuse unlikely.

Metabolic alkalosis following vomiting may cause urinary potassium loss. This occurs because the presence of bicarbonate anion in tubular fluid increases luminal negative charge and the movement of potassium down its electrochemical gradient out of tubular cells is increased.

After consideration of these diagnoses a few patients, of whom this man is an example, remain with unexplained urinary potassium loss. They are often categorized as *'Bartter's Syndrome'* although it is unlikely that they are a homogeneous group particularly as the clinical presentation varies from a severe illness with thirst, polyuria, dehydration, weakness and, in infants, failure to thrive to an asymptomatic presentation in adult life. A family history is common and a variety of associated features may be present: hypomagnesaemia, acidification defects, hypercalcuria and radiographic abnormalities (nephrocalcinosis, dilatation of the urinary tract).

Typically patients with the syndrome have a high plasma renin and are resistant to the pressor effect of infused angiotensin. Renal biopsy reveals hyperplasia of the juxtaglomerular apparatus and may show tubular vacuolation. The juxtaglomerular changes may be found in other hyperreninaemic conditions such as Addison's disease and laxative or diuretic abuse and are not diagnostic.

The mechanism of hypotension and angiotensin resistance is uncertain. In the syndrome there is hyperplasia of medullary interstitial cells and increased urinary excretion of prostaglandin E2 and of 6-keto-PGF1α, the principal metabolite of prostacyclin. One possibility is that these prostaglandins reach the blood stream and lower vascular tone. The significance of abnormal rates of sodium and potassium flux across red cell membranes in some patients is uncertain.

Treatment has been attempted with potassium supplements, spironolactone, amiloride, propranolol and adrenalectomy, but correction of potassium depletion is seldom achieved. The failure of adrenalectomy to correct hypokalaemia indicates that hyper-aldosteronism is not the principal cause of potassium loss.

Therapy with prostaglandin synthetase inhibitors, usually indomethacin, causes both clinical and biochemical improvement, although long-term correction of potassium depletion is unusual. The combination of prostaglandin synthetase inhibitors and potassium supplements is now the treatment of choice for most cases. Occasional patients are hypomagnesaemic and may respond to magnesium supplements. In this patient, who has no symptoms, specific therapy is not essential.

The prognosis with treatment is not known.

Case 30

Mr J. S.

A 71-year-old retired butcher was referred from another hospital for investigation of nephrotic syndrome. He had been in good health for most of his life but had lost 12 kg in weight over the last year, with increasing lethargy and loss of appetite. He also experienced dizzy spells on standing and tingling and pain in his hands in bed at night. He had developed ankle oedema over the past two months and 'easy bruising' of his legs with purpura. There was a family history of diabetes but none of TB or renal disease. On examination he was a tense man with obvious weight loss and purpura on his legs. Pulse was irregular 90/minute, blood pressure 130/85 mmHg supine and 60/20 mmHg with no increase in pulse rate, when erect. The JVP was normal and the chest was clear but there was ankle oedema. There was three fingers non-tender hepatomegaly but no splenomegaly. Neurological examination revealed impaired sensation of the first three fingers of both hands.

Results showed Hb 12.1 g/dl, WCC 8.0 × $10^9/\ell$, platelets 324 × $10^9/\ell$, ESR 24 mm/hour, urea 7 mmol/ℓ (42 mg/100 ml), creatinine 100 μmol/ℓ (1.1 mg/100 ml), K 3.8 mmol/ℓ, albumin 23 g/ℓ, blood sugar 6.0 mmol/ℓ (108 mg/100 ml), 10 g of unselective proteinuria/day and a creatinine clearance of 95 ml/minute. ECG showed right bundle branch block with ventricular ectopics. CXR, barium enema and meal were normal. Ultrasound of the liver showed diffuse enlargement while on IVU the kidneys were normal size. A WR and Mantoux were negative as was a Kveim test, SCAT, Latex and ANF.

Questions

1. What are the possible diagnoses?
2. Would a renal biopsy help in diagnosis and management?

Comment

This is a case of nephrotic syndrome with evidence of systemic disease. As in all cases of nephrotic syndrome, and most of renal failure the most useful diagnostic investigation is the renal biopsy. In this case a biopsy would give a descriptive label of the renal lesion but may not reveal the underlying systemic disease.

Symptoms and signs supporting a systemic disease rather than localized renal pathology are anorexia with marked weight loss, hepatomegaly, purpura, postural hypotension without tachycardia (indicative of autonomic neuropathy), carpal tunnel syndrome and an abnormal ECG. (Hepatomegaly can occasionally occur in nephrotic syndrome because of increased plasma protein metabolism.)

Carcinomatosis is possible in view of his age and history, although a chest x-ray and barium series were normal. A variety of malignancies have been associated with membranous glomerulonephritis and carcinoma of the lung with a Henoch–Schönlein type syndrome. Minimal change glomerulonephritis has been reported in Hodgkin's disease supporting the role of the lymphocyte in the aetiology of this lesion.

There is no evidence of a connective tissue disorder from serology results, although it is recognized that symptoms can pre-date positive serology.

Other possible systemic disorders, such as diabetes, TB, syphilis and sarcoid are excluded on investigation.

In this case the renal biopsy was positive for amyloid, showing under polarized light birefringence with Congo Red in the mesangia, extending along the basement membrane.

Amyloid occurs in three pathological types, as a *primary disease*, or associated with multiple myeloma, as a *complication of a chronic disease* (such as rheumatoid arthritis or infection) and as the rare and geographically distinct *familial neuropathies* (e.g. Portuguese).

In this case electrophoresis of the urine showed predominant albuminuria but on immunoelectrophoresis a Lambda paraprotein band was detected. Bone marrow contained 10% atypical plasma cells although there was no evidence of skeletal involvement. Therefore the diagnosis is amyloid with multiple myeloma.

The clinical classification of amyloid by organ involvement has become outdated and unsatisfactory as a biochemical basis of the disease is defined.

All amyloid consists of two proteins. P substance protein is present in all types comprising 5% of the total amyloid volume. The second protein can be of three types, either fragments of immuno-globulin light chain (AL), AA protein or pre-albumin. In 'primary' amyloid and that associated with myeloma, light chain fragments are found (AL) in secondary amyloid AA protein is present, while in the familial amyloidoses, pre-albumin is the second protein constituent.

Primary amyloid and amyloid with myeloma occur most frequently in men in their mid 60s presenting with weakness, fatigue, weight loss, oedema, bruising, paraesthesia, syncope, voice changes or carpal tunnel syndrome. Enlargement of the liver or tongue are often found and purpura may be present in face, neck and eyelids. Oedema suggests a nephrotic syndrome (occurring in 30% of patients) or heart failure (occurring in 25%). Ninety per cent of patients have proteinuria, with renal failure of varying degrees in 50%. A paraprotein is found in urine or serum in 90% of patients and is most frequently of the Lambda subtype.

The severity of the nephrotic syndrome does not correlate with extent of amyloid deposition. Rarer renal complications are the Fanconi syndrome and renal vein thrombosis.

The mean survival after diagnosis is a year, with cardiac failure and arrhythmias accounting for the majority of deaths and renal failure as the second most important cause.

Treatment is unsatisfactory though cytotoxics (melphalan and prednisolone) may help. Colchicine, vitamin C and dimethyl sulphoxide (DMSO) are under investigation. Renal transplantation can prevent death from renal failure though amyloid can recur in the graft. The patient described progressed and died of amyloid cardiac involvement.

Case 31

Mrs Y. T.

This 26-year-old woman attended the outpatient department with a single episode of dysuria and urinary frequency of 5 days' duration. Aged 5 years, she had been investigated for recurrent right-sided abdominal pain and a urinary infection was diagnosed. An IVU showed an apical scar in the left kidney with no abnormality of the outflow tract on this side. The right kidney and outflow tract were normal. Micturating cystogram showed vesicoureteric reflux on the left. The bladder emptied normally. Blood pressure was 115/80 mmHg, creatinine clearance 20 ml/minute/m^2 surface area.

She received regular antibiotic therapy for 4 years, the urine remained sterile, serial plain abdominal x-rays showed no further scarring and steady growth of both kidneys. Aged 10 repeat micturating cystogram showed no evidence of reflux and throughout adolescence she had remained well with no urinary symptoms.

The present symptoms were disturbing her as she wished for a pregnancy and sought advice in this regard also. On examination blood pressure was 115/75 mmHg. No skeletal or neurological abnormalities and no abdominal tenderness were found.

Investigations: serum creatinine 90 μmol/ℓ, creatinine clearance 100 ml/minute (70 ml/minute/m^2 surface area), MSU — 5 pus cells/ high powered field, pure growth of *E.coli* greater than 10^5 organisms/ml, no proteinuria. IVU — apical polar scar left kidney, both kidneys otherwise normal in size and shape. Both outflow tracts normal, as was the bladder.

Questions

1. What treatment is required?
2. What advice should she be given regarding pregnancy?

Comment

The urine infection may be treated with trimethoprim alone. There is continuing debate about the length of time for which therapy is required. In an uncomplicated case, an isolated infection may be cured by 'natural defences' or by a short course of effective chemotherapy (1–5 days).

Mrs Y. T. had established non-progressive pyelonephritis, the result of urine infections before the age of 5 years. At this early age, but much less frequently later, urine infection may cause renal scarring especially if there is ureteric reflux. The early recognition, prompt and continued therapy and careful follow-up had ensured that renal damage, sustained in early life, was arrested. Renal growth was protected by eliminating infection and, as often occurs, the mild vesicoureteric reflux of early life, ceased as the urinary tracts matured, a process made more likely in the absence of urinary infection.

After treatment with trimethoprim for 5 days, the urine became sterile and remained so on regular testing every 2 months over the next 18 months. The excellent renal function now recorded, the absence of hypertension and the eventually sterilized urine are all factors pointing to the present health of the renal parenchyma. The development of an isolated infection in adult life is not relevant to the previous history and it is unlikely that, the lower urinary tract being normal as in this case, further renal damage will ensue.

Uncomplicated pregnancy can be expected. Care should be taken that the blood pressure remains normal and that infection does not complicate the pregnancy, but neither of these complications is more likely to occur than in any other healthy young woman.

It is noteworthy that it has often been thought that a previous history of parenchymal renal disease is a contraindication to pregnancy. There is now ample evidence that where such a disease has ceased and renal function is stable, a more optimistic approach is possible.

Case 32

Mr J. H.

A 50-year-old gardener was brought to casualty at 10.00 am complaining of stomach pains and vomiting. At 10.00 pm the previous night he had swallowed 20 ml of a concentrated weedkiller which he had obtained from work. In the previous three months since his wife had left him, and his children had stopped visiting him, he had taken two overdoses of aspirin. On examination he showed little emotion but was not physically distressed. He had ulceration of his mouth. His chest was clear, pulse 90 beats/minute regular and blood pressure 200/105 mmHg. There was epigastric tenderness. Routine urinalysis showed blood + albumin + + and blood tests, urea 2.8 mmol/ℓ (17 mg/100 ml), Na 139 mmol/ℓ, Hb 16.3 g/dl, WCC 17.1 × $10^9/\ell$, platelets 212 × $10^9/\ell$, pH 7.52 PO_2 95 mmHg, PCO_2 31.5 mmHg, actual bicarbonate 23.5 mmol/ℓ, base excess +2 mmol/ℓ. Chest x-ray was normal.

Questions

1. What is the diagnosis?
2. What is the treatment?
3. What is the prognosis and complications?

Comment

This depressed but orientated man, at his third attempt at suicide had chosen a method which he thought was certain to be effective. The two weedkillers to which there is ready access are paraquat and sodium chlorate. He chose paraquat, a weedkiller available in low concentration (25 g/kg) in Pathclear and Weedol and also for professional use as a highly concentrated form (200 g/ℓ) Gramoxone, Dextrone, Dexuron, Gramanol. The diagnosis is rapidly confirmed by a screening test on urine or gastric washings. The natural history of the disease is of progressive respiratory failure caused by interstitial and intra-alveolar fibrosis of the lungs with a high mortality. In more severe cases as here, early acute renal failure occurs. This may recover in 7 to 10 days, only for the patient to die of the respiratory failure, for which once established no treatment is available.

Treatment, which must be urgent, is aimed at removing paraquat both from the bowel and the blood, and possibly the tissues. Once paraquat has been absorbed from the gut it is readily taken up by the lung where it causes most damage and is difficult to remove, bound to the tissues. Unless treatment is effected rapidly (preferably within 4 hours of ingestion) recovery is unlikely.

The stomach should be washed out and 1 ℓ of 15% Fuller's Earth (to absorb paraquat) with 200 ml 20% mannitol in water (as a purgative) instilled. Sodium or magnesium sulphate can be used as alternatives to mannitol and should be continued until they are present in the stool. A poison centre should be contacted for urgent advice on further treatment. Serum levels of paraquat may be helpful but because of the avid tissue absorption do not reflect the total body content after the first 12 hours. The difficulty is in deciding which patients have taken enough paraquat to warrant haemoperfusion but not too much to be inevitably fatal so needing symptomatic treatment only. The Gramoxone type preparation is concentrated and a mouthful is often fatal. However, Weedol poisoning is less serious as few people ingest a sufficiently large dose. It may be cured by purgation alone. Haemoperfusion removes more paraquat than haemodialysis and energetic treatment within the first 12 hours continued for 10–15 hours on successive days may be lifesaving.

Once the lung fibrosis has occurred and arterial PO_2 begins to fall it is important to withhold oxygen therapy as this can potentiate the lung damage.

Mouth and oesophageal ulceration is common with the more concentrated preparations.

In our patient rapidly progressive renal failure required dialysis by the third day but renal function began improving by the tenth day. The arterial PO_2 fell on the third day and assisted ventilation was required. However it became impossible to oxygenate his lungs and he died as a consequence of lung fibrosis 12 days after admission.

Note: Haemoperfusion is a method of passing blood through a column of activated charcoal which absorbs the poison but also results in a fall in the platelet and white cell count.

Case 33

Mr C. S.

A 37-year-old lorry driver was transferred from a district general hospital for further investigation and management. Over the previous 2 months he had suffered generalized lassitude and occasional night sweats. Two weeks earlier he had noticed smoky urine progressing to gross painless haematuria. There had been a decrease in urine volume to total anuria for the last 4 days. There was nausea and vomiting with generalized aching in his muscles and lower limbs, orthopnoea and haemoptysis. For many years he had lumbar disc pain and regularly took large quantities of compound analgesics. As a child he had a cervical lymph node removed surgically but he had not received any antituberculous chemotherapy. He had not had any recent sore throats and there was no family history of renal disease or deafness.

He was admitted to his local hospital where his blood urea was 51 mmol/ℓ (306 mg/100 ml), creatinine 1850 μmol/ℓ (20.9 mg/100 ml) and potassium 7.2 mmol/ℓ, so urgent peritoneal dialysis was commenced. On transfer to us he was orientated and apyrexial. Pulse 90 beats/minute regular, blood pressure 150/90 mmHg with a pan-systolic murmur audible all over the precordium, JVP was raised 5 cm with sacral and ankle oedema and a few basal crepitations in the chest. There was no evidence of vasculitis. Results showed Hb 10.1 g/dl (normochromic normocytic), WCC 11.2 × 10⁹/ℓ (with a normal differential), platelets 355 × 10⁹/ℓ and ESR 77 mm/ hour. Blood urea was 39.5 mmol/ℓ (237 mg/100 ml), creatinine 1480 μmol/ℓ (16.7 mg/100 ml), albumin 26 g/ℓ, phosphate 3.0 mmol/ℓ (9.63 mg/100 ml), complement studies, ANF and ASO titres and coagulation studies normal.

Chest x-ray showed an enlarged heart with diffuse shadowing of both lung fields compatible with alveolar oedema. The kidneys were normal in size on tomography and a renal biopsy showed an aggressive glomerulonephritis with 100% crescents and extensive fibrin deposits. There was no evidence of arteritis.

Questions

1. What are the possible diagnoses?
2. What other tests are needed to make a diagnosis?
3. What treatment is possible?

Comment

This is a case of acute renal failure caused by crescentic glomerulonephritis. The 'red herrings' in the history are the analgesic consumption which can produce analgesic nephropathy, but not a crescentic nephritis and previous tuberculosis which may result in renal parenchymatous disease and possibly chronic obstructive renal failure. Crescentic glomerular nephritis is either idiopathic or secondary to a systemic vasculitis such as a polyarteritis, Henoch–Schönlein syndrome or systemic lupus erythematosus. In this case there was no evidence of a vasculitis clinically or on biopsy however it may be diagnosable only at post mortem. Henoch–Schönlein nephritis usually has a purpuric rash and glomerular IgA deposits and a negative ANF does not support a diagnosis of SLE.

A small clue in the history is the haemoptysis. Although he has a possible cause in his fluid overload he continued to have haemoptysis when his fluid balance was corrected. The combination of haemoptysis and crescentic glomerulonephritis gives the full Goodpasture's syndrome. This is a rare disease, but is important as an experimental model and because successful treatment is now available. The diagnosis is confirmed by measuring circulatory anti Glomerular Basement Membrane (anti GBM) antibodies and demonstrating linear staining of immunoglobulin (usually IgG but rarely IgG and M) on glomerular basement membranes by immunofluorescence. The pattern of immunoglobulin deposition can become distorted and no longer linear as glomerular damage proceeds.

The dual involvement of lung and kidney is thought to be due to the cross reaction of an antibody to lung and glomerular basement membranes — linear deposits of immunoglobulins can be demonstrated in lung biopsy specimens though recent evidence suggests that the lung antibody may be different. The spectrum of Goodpasture's syndrome (anti GBM disease) is wider than the classically florid form with lung purpurae and nephritis. There may be mild chronic nephritis without lung involvement as well as primary pulmonary haemosiderosis with little renal damage. The levels of circulating antibody do not correlate with the severity of the pulmonary involvement. The aetiology of the disease is uncertain although viral infections and exposure to hydrocarbon solvents may play a part in both initiating the disease and in recurrence. Ninety per cent of patients possess the HLA antigen DR2 and prognosis is poorer if this is accompanied by the HLA antigen B7.

Treatment is aimed at either modifying the disease by immunosuppression and plasmaphoresis sometimes combined with nephrectomy which is said to ameliorate the pulmonary disease, or renal replacement by dialysis and transplantation. Nephrectomy, once popular, has little effect on the natural history. In a few cases urgent plasmaphoresis combined with immunosuppression halts and reverses the decline in renal function but has little benefit in the anuric patient. Plasmaphoresis may be lifesaving in fulminant pulmonary haemorrhage regardless of the state of the renal disease. If the disease is suspected urgent renal biopsy and anti GBM antibody assay is indicated in order to commence potentially successful treatment.

Transplantation should be delayed until levels of anti GBM antibody are within the normal range to prevent recurrence in the graft.

Our patient had raised levels of anti GBM antibodies but in view of his anuria and already severely damaged kidney, neither immunosuppression or plasmaphoresis were thought justified. He was dialysed and subsequently received successfully a cadaver kidney when his anti GBM antibody levels were within the normal range.

Case 34

Mr R. E.

A 42-year-old company director had an 18-year history of recurrent episodes of renal colic, each of which began as a constant bilateral upper lumbar ache lasting for a few weeks and culminating in a typical attack of severe colicky loin pain, radiating to one or other groin. Some hours later the pain would spontaneously resolve and he would pass a variable number of small spiculated stones. He had never been aware of haematuria. Currently he has about 3 attacks per year. Apart from requiring opiates for the pain he has required no other medication and has otherwise been a fit healthy man with no significant social, family or past medical history. His elderly parents and older siblings were alive and well. On physical examination he had a normal blood pressure and no cardiovascular, respiratory or neurological abnormality. Abdominal examination did not reveal any palpable renal masses or loin tenderness. Investigations: Hb 16.4 g/dl; ESR 5 mm/hour; WCC 6.4 × 10^9/ℓ; plasma urea 4.5 mmol/ℓ (27 mg/100 ml); plasma creatinine 73 μmol/ℓ (0.8 mg/100 ml); plasma calcium 2.3 mmol/ℓ; phosphate 0.7 mmol/ℓ; plasma urate 0.35 mmol/ℓ; serum PTH normal; astrup normal; thyroxine 110 nmol/ℓ (normal 55–130); MSU, no cells, no growth; urine acidification (short acid load test) reached a pH of 5; 24 hour urine protein 0.09 g; 24 hour urine calcium excretion 6 mmol (normal 2.5 to 7.5); urine phosphate oxalate and urate excretion, normal; urine chromatogram showed a normal amino acid pattern; radiographs of hands revealed no evidence of hyperparathyroidism; the plain film before IVU showed a small cluster of calculi within the upper pyramids of both kidneys which were normal in size. With contrast, streaks of medium were seen which appeared to pass back from the otherwise well-defined calyces, with small pools of contrast surrounding the calculi, and collections of dye appearing separately in other pyramids (*see* p. 141).

Questions

1. What is the diagnosis?
2. If presented with the plain film only, what is the differential diagnosis?

Comment

The radiographic findings are those of medullary sponge kidney (MSK). This condition, a congenital abnormality of uncertain pathogenesis, is characterized pathologically by small dilatations of the collecting system within the renal medulla. In any one individual these 'cystic' lesions may be localized to one part of one kidney, or scattered throughout both kidneys. Clinical attention is usually drawn to the patient because of renal colic, frequently with passage of a stone, haematuria or upper urinary tract infection. Plain radiographs of the abdomen commonly reveal a few to a dozen or more calcified opacities, typically located in groups. These are usually calcium phosphate stones, found within the cysts, but interstitial intramedullary deposition may also be found. The differential diagnosis of such nephrocalcinosis includes causes of hypercalcaemia for example sarcoidosis, vitamin D intoxication and hyperparathyroidism as well as idiopathic renal tubular acidosis and tuberculosis. With intravenous urography the diagnosis is usually obvious. The cysts fill with dye before the pelvis opacifies and there is delayed emptying of these dilatations. Furthermore, the dye surrounds the stones indicating that they are intracystic. This excludes the other causes of calcinosis.

GFR is usually normal, even after many years of follow-up, providing obstruction or infection have not resulted in tissue destruction. In some patients minor defects in concentrating and acidification abilities are reported, but it is debated whether these are primary or secondary manifestations of the disorder.

The condition may become apparent at any time from childhood to late adult life and only rarely does it have a familial inheritance. A few reports comment on the association between MSK and primary hyperparathyroidism. It may be that the latter condition simply unmasks the former, which otherwise would have remained silent. In general, MSK is thought to predispose to stone formation and therefore it would seem prudent in symptomatic patients to give dietary advice in order to avoid excessive calcium and oxalate ingestion, and to maintain a satisfactory fluid intake.

A totally separate condition, which unfortunately sounds similar, medullary cystic disease, should not be confused with MSK. Apart from the finding of cystic lesions in the medulla, the clinical features are quite distinct. In medullary cystic disease, the cysts are always bilateral and stone formation is absent. Most commonly the cysts are part of a non-functioning nephron; these may develop as diverticulae of the distal collecting system, and grow to exceed 1 cm diameter. The initiating event in the production of such a lesion is unknown.

In medullary cystic disease, there is frequently a family history of the disease, or of 'renal failure'. The inheritance appears to be autosomal recessive, although the dominant mode is also postulated, the latter appearing to be more common when presentation is in adult life. Other features that serve to distinguish it from MSK includes the absence of nephrocalcinosis and the failure to demonstrate the cysts on urography. The IVU usually reveals small shrunken kidneys in the later stages of the disease. Corticomedullary cysts may be demonstrated by angiography. This condition frequently results in terminal renal failure in adolescence and early adulthood. An interesting, though not universal, finding is the inability of the kidneys to retain sodium which, unless adequate supplementation is taken, leads to postural hypotension, more particularly as function becomes impaired.

Case 35

Mr S. W.

You are asked by the urologists to see a 20-year-old single newsagent with a history of renal calculi. Four years previously he had an episode of pyelitis and epididymitis and subsequently he passed a small stone per urethra. Following this he was investigated and was found on IVU to have a small poorly functioning scarred right kidney with a faintly radio-opaque staghorn calculus within its pelvis. A right nephrectomy was performed and histologically there were pyelonephritic changes with calculi within the kidney though no evidence of medullary sponge kidney. His presentation this time was of left-sided renal colic and anuria. The left ureter had become blocked with a faintly radio-opaque stone which required pyelo-ureterolithotomy. He was an obese young man with no brothers or sisters though an uncle had 'kidney stones' but he was unsure of what type they were. Examination was normal with a blood pressure of 140/80 mmHg. Investigations 10 days post operatively showed: sodium 140 mmol/ℓ, potassium 4.5 mmol/ℓ, urea 7.6 mmol/ℓ (46 mg/100 ml), creatinine 95 μmol/ℓ (1.1 mg/100 ml), chloride 100 mmol/ℓ, blood sugar 5.2 mmol/ℓ (94 mg/100 ml), calcium 2.35 mmol/ℓ (9.6 mg/100 ml), phosphate 0.92 mmol/ℓ (2.95 mg/100 ml), alkaline phos-phatase 60 IU/ℓ, urate 0.39 mmol/ℓ (6.5 mg/100 ml). An acid load test with ammonium chloride produced a minimum urine pH of 4.8. A 24 hour urine showed insignificant proteinuria and 6.5 mmol (26.1 mg) calcium. An MSU was sterile.

The problem, therefore, is of a young man with recurrent stones and the possibility of irreversible damage to his remaining kidney.

Questions

1. What further tests need to be done?
2. What is the probable diagnosis?
3. What is the treatment?

Comment

In deciding what further tests could be done one should consider the possible diagnoses and aim to confirm or exclude them. The first clue is the relatively low radiodensity of the staghorn calculus and stone indicating a low calcium content. Stones of calcium oxalate and phosphate are densely radio-opaque whilst those of xanthine and uric acid are radiolucent. Cystine and magnesium-ammonium-phosphate stones are moderately opaque. A further point against any high calcium stones is the normal urinary calcium of 6.5 mmol/day (260 mg/day, normal 2.5–7.5 mmol or 100–300 mg/day). To confirm the stone constituents chemical analysis should be performed on the material removed at pyeloureterolithotomy. In this case the stone was virtually pure cystine (with a slight coating of calcium phosphate).

The diagnosis of cystinuria can be made with a urine test for cystine which in this case was strongly positive with 5 mmol/24 hours (400 mg) cystine (normal 0.2–0.63 mmol/24 hours, 16–50 mg/24 hours). The more specialized test of urinary amino acid chromatography showed a gross excess of cystine, lysine, ornithine and arginine, the basic amino acids. These share a common resorption pathway at the luminal surface of the proximal tubule.

The second clue to diagnosis is the evidence of a possible inherited condition; an uncle also had renal calculi. Cystinuria usually has an autosomal recessive inheritance, the homozygote being the stone producer (especially in males). There are two subtypes of this disease depending on whether there is a urinary excess of four amino acids (cystine, lysine, ornithine and arginine) or just two (cystine and lysine). The basic defect is an abnormality in proximal tubular transport of these amino acids. There is no evidence of other proximal tubular disorders (renal glycosuria, hypophosphataemia or hypouricaemia).

Cystine stones are rare and account for only 1% of renal calculi but are important in that treatment can prevent their occurrence which can result in renal damage. The treatment is aimed at ensuring that the unabsorbed cystine in the urine is at a low enough concentration to prevent saturation and stone formation, usually below 2.4 mmol (200 mg)/ℓ. The most important and often difficult part of the treatment is the education of the patient to drink at least three (preferably five) litres of fluid per day. It is essential that this volume is spread out during the day. The patient should be trained to wake up at night to pass urine and drink half to one litre of fluid.

Cystine is more soluble in alkali than acid therefore sodium bicarbonate (10 g/day) may be used to keep the urine pH between 7 and 7.5.

A further adjuvant to therapy is D-penicillamine at a dose of 1.5 g/day. This forms a soluble cystine-disulphide complex so reducing the chance of cystine precipitation in the urine.

Stones already formed may be 'washed away' with adequate treatment when the urine cystine concentration is reduced consistently as described. Treatment is continued for life and the state of stone formation monitored by regular abdominal x-ray.

In the case described, despite several periods of in hospital 'training', lack of compliance occurred at home with regular new stone formation.

Case 36

Mr I. M.

A 31-year-old chemical engineer had viral meningitis 7 years previously. He had been well until developing 'hay fever' for the first time 2 years ago. Later that year he experienced sharp right-sided pleuritic pain. He was investigated in hospital where chest x-rays, electrocardiogram, intravenous urogram and barium swallow and meal were all normal. No definite diagnosis was made and he was given no treatment. Two months later he developed a constant pain on the bridge of his nose with rhinorrhoea, which failed to resolve with antibiotics. One year ago while on a business trip to America he noticed pain in his calves and ankles with swelling, erythema and a purpuric rash. He was dyspnoeic with chest discomfort, although no pleuritic pain and a non-productive cough. He had blood stained rhinorrhoea. He was admitted to hospital where his temperature was 39.5 °C. Blood pressure 140/80 mmHg, pulse 110 regular with no lymphadenopathy and no focal signs in the chest. The nasal septum was injected and scarred with a perforation. Ward testing of urine showed blood $++$ and protein $++$. A midstream urine showed granular casts with 100 RBC per high power field. Other results: Hb 10.4 g/dl, MCV 79 fl, slight polychromasia, reticulocyte count 0.8%, WCC $11.8 \times 10^9/\ell$ (62% neutrophils, 30% lymphocytes, 8% monocytes), platelets $600 \times 10^9/\ell$, direct Coombs' test negative. Na 135 mmol/ℓ, K 4.4 mmol/ℓ, urea 8.0 mmol/ℓ (48 mg/100 ml), creatinine 100 μmol/ℓ (1.1 mg/100 ml), albumin 35 g/ℓ, urinary protein 1.7 g/24 hours. Antinuclear factor negative, cryoglobulins negative, immunoelectrophoresis showed a polyclonal increase in IgG and IgM. Sputum culture grew normal flora and blood cultures were negative. Chest x-ray showed multiple nodular lesions in the right lung with cavitation in some without hilar lymphadenopathy. Sinus x-rays showed clouding of the left frontal sinus.

Questions

1. What is the diagnosis?
2. How can you confirm it?
3. What is the treatment and prognosis?

Comment

The diagnosis is Wegener's granulomatosis which was confirmed by nasal and open lung biopsy. Both showed severely inflamed muscular blood vessels occluded by inflammatory cells and thrombus reaction with granulomata containing multinucleated giant cells.

His condition deteriorated rapidly, within 2 weeks of admission urea was 30 mmol/ℓ (180 mg/100 ml), creatinine 670 μmol/ℓ (7.5. mg/100 ml) and albumin dropping to 17 g/ℓ. He was therefore started on cyclophosphamide 150 mg/day. The chest x-ray changes cleared, urea returned to 8 mmol/ℓ (48 mg/100 ml) and creatinine to 265 μmol/ℓ (3 mg/100 ml) but proteinuria of 10 g/24 hours persisted. Renal biopsy was performed which showed sclerosis of 22 of 37 glomeruli obtained with widespread crescent formation. The remaining glomeruli showed a variable increase in mesangial cells. There were no granulomata and no arteritic lesions in the biopsy specimen. Renal function declined and the patient eventually required haemodialysis 1 year later.

Wegener's granulomatosis is a rare disease more common in men (3:2), being classified in the polyarteritic group of disorders (*see Table 36.1*).

Goodpasture's syndrome is the other pulmonary renal syndrome to consider in the differential diagnosis.

Cases of Wegener's granulomatosis do not always have renal involvement although its occurrence implies a worse prognosis. The renal damage may not be due to the arteritis itself but to circulating immune complexes being deposited in the kidney. Raised serum levels of complexes have been found in active disease and a few patients have responded to plasmaphoresis.

The natural history of the disease is of relapses often associated with infection, the upper respiratory tract signs and symptoms preceding further renal damage.

Treatment is with cyclophosphamide with or without steroids and possibly plasmaphoresis to induce remission and then maintenance with azathioprine with or without steroids.

The use of cyclophosphamide has improved the prognosis and cure is now possible. Renal function may continue to decline without other evidence of active disease due to the extensive initial damage and progressive scarring as illustrated in this case.

Table 36.1   Classification – PAN type vasculitis

	PAN	Allergic Granulomatous Disease	Hyper-sensitivity Vasculitis	Wegener's Granulomatosis
Vessels	Small and medium vessels. Bifurcation points	Diffuse extravascular granuloma	Small arteries and veins	Small and medium arteries
Signs symptoms	Severe hypertension	History of asthma	Skin purpura (precipitation by drugs)	URTI Sinusitis (Hypertension is rare)
Organs affected	Kidneys + + Gut Liver Coronary arteries (Not lungs)	Lungs (eosinophilia in sputum and blood)	Skin Lungs Kidneys	Nasal septum Lungs Kidneys

Case 37

Mr L. M.

At the age of 30 years, Mr L. M. started work as a foundryman and was later employed as a 'pourer' involved in the production of copper and cadmium alloys. Due to the known association between exposure to cadmium fumes and development of respiratory disease, a prospective study of employees in this foundry was undertaken. By 1962, within 2 years of the first exposure, his urine cadmium excretion was recorded at 730 µg/ℓ, but proteinuria was absent. In 1967, the Factories Act made cadmium poisoning a notifiable disease, and in 1968 this patient was moved to another job which prevented further exposure. Urine cadmium concentration fell abruptly, but continued at about 25 µg/ℓ, with a quantitative protein excretion of approximately 1 g in 24 hours. Plasma urea remained normal over the next decade. He was fully investigated in 1980 and no other informative clinical history was forthcoming. Examination was entirely unremarkable, but the following results were obtained: Hb 16.2 g/dl; PCV 48%; platelets 212 × 10^9/ℓ; ESR 11 mm/hour; plasma urea 5.9 mmol/ℓ (35 mg/100 ml); plasma creatinine 140 µmol/ℓ (1.6 mg/100 ml); plasma albumin 43 g/ℓ; serum urate 0.19

mmol/ℓ; serum immunoglobulins and electrophoresis and complement profile, normal; SCAT, Latex, ANF and SLE cell tests, all negative; glucose tolerance test, normal; 24 hour urine protein 1.3 g; urine electrophoresis revealed albumin, α_2 and β_2 globulin and excess β_2 microglobulin was present; urine chromatogram demonstrated generalized aminoaciduria; repeated testing of urine was positive for glucose; urine osmolality after an overnight fast, 884 mmol/kg; acid load test produced a urine of pH 4.9; IVU, normal; renal biopsy showed 2 of 10 glomeruli to be sclerosed and the others normal by light microscopy, with negative immunofluorescence, but mild tubular changes with swollen epithelial cells and some focal degeneration. The interstitium was unremarkable.

Questions

1. From the information supplied where in the nephron is the functional abnormality associated with cadmium nephropathy?
2. What lesions are associated with such other metal 'poisonings' as lead, mercury, copper and gold?

Comment

Patients with cadmium poisoning were amongst the first studied in the delineation of a 'tubular' proteinuria as distinct from the pattern of urine proteins found in glomerular disease. Detection of protein with Albustix and the salicylsulphonic acid test will be positive, but boiling tests may be negative. Commonly, with tubular disease from any cause, only 1–2 g of protein are found in a 24 hour urine collection, and although up to 50% may be albumin (MW 68 000) most of the rest is of proteins with molecular weights in the 20 000–30 000 range. This finding is explained by the concept that even with a normal glomerulus, small amounts of high and low molecular weight proteins appear in the urinary space. With intact non-selective tubular resorptive processes, less than 200–300 mg of protein are excreted daily. In tubular malfunction however much of the filtered protein load remains unabsorbed and appears in the urine. Patients with a glomerular protein leak may excrete over 20 g of protein in the urine each day and much the greatest contribution is from albumin. The urine also contains variable amounts of higher molecular weight proteins. With this patient the pattern of proteinuria, particularly the finding of β_2 microglobulin, a protein with a molecular weight of 10 000, in the urine, indicates tubular damage. The ability to achieve a urine pH of less than 5.3 and a concentration in excess of 800 mmol/kg indicates functional integrity of the distal tubule, whereas the appearance of renal glycosuria and generalized aminoaciduria in conjunction with a low plasma urate (and by inference a high urine urate clearance) tends to localize the lesion to the proximal tubule. Interstitial abnormalities are also reported in biopsies of patients with cadmium poisoning, but were not present in Mr L. M.

Cadmium exposure usually occurs in smelting plants. The element is a component of alloys particularly valuable in the manufacture of engine parts, and was formerly added to solder and specialized wires. Acute ingestion leads to a severe, but rapidly self-limiting, episode of gastrointestinal symptoms and acute massive inhalation of cadmium fumes results in acute pneumonitis and occasionally death. The more common problem is that of chronic inhalation which causes emphysema and tubular protein-uria. Deposition in liver, and development of abnormal liver function tests is recorded, and anosmia, due to mucosal damage is said to occur. In Japan, cadmium poisoning is associated with the development of painful osteomalacia known as 'ouch ouch' disease. With consistent exposure, relatively high urine excretion rates are obtained, but on cessation of that exposure elimination of cadmium may be prolonged at relatively low levels for many years. Renal failure is rare and probably only occurs with protracted and excessive exposure, at which time a fall in concentrating ability suggests distal tubule or interstitial involvement as well.

The evidence for implicating other metals in the genesis of renal lesions is controversial. It is believed that acute lead poisoning leads to tubular damage, with aminoaciduria, glycosuria and proteinuria and that chronic exposure results in interstitial fibrosis. The glomerular changes seen with chronic exposure may be secondary to vascular involvement.

Mercury has long been associated with the development of a nephrotic syndrome noted when it was so commonly used as the earliest potent diuretic. More recently its use in skin-lightening creams has been implicated in the development of a glomerular lesion. The pathogenesis remains obscure but here, and in the nephropathy associated with gold therapy, it has been suggested that primary tubular damage results in the release of antigens which precipitate an immune complex glomerulonephritis. Other reports incriminate mercury in the appearance of a Fanconi's syndrome and of a necrotizing lesion of the renal tubules.

There is a well recognized association between copper overload in Wilson's disease and proximal tubule damage manifested by generalized aminoaciduria. Other metals such as bismuth, silver and antimony may be associated to a greater or lesser degree with renal damage.

Case 38

Mr J. S.

A 34-year-old electrical engineer was found to have a blood pressure of 190/110 mmHg at an examination performed on behalf of an insurance company. Aortic systolic and diastolic murmurs were noted, and protein was detected in the urine. Salient features in the history included an attack of rheumatic fever at the age of 14 years during which he was confined to bed for 6 months, and the death of his father at the age of 38 years from an unknown cause. An intravenous urogram confirmed the diagnosis of polycystic renal disease, which had been suspected after palpation of the abdomen. Plasma urea and creatinine were raised and treatment for his hypertension was commenced.

Over the next 4 years, his renal function deteriorated and he required a short period of intermittent peritoneal dialysis, together with propranolol and hydralazine to control his blood pressure, a 30 g selected, high biological value protein diet (in conjunction with vitamin supplements) to try to minimize azotaemia, and aluminium hydroxide taken with meals in order to decrease gastrointestinal phosphate absorption. He was eventually trained for home dialysis. Fifteen months later he received a cadaver graft but this failed to function and was removed after 4 weeks, histology showing acute rejection. He returned to haemodialysis, and full time employment.

Two years after restarting haemodialysis he became aware of some difficulty in speaking, 'unable to get the words out', particularly after a dialysis session. He also commented that his memory was poor and that he was making simple errors in his job. Formal psychological testing confirmed a mild organic memory deficit and an EEG showed features consistent with the presumptive diagnosis. Bone biopsy revealed osteomalacia; indeed, he had been complaining of widespread bone pains and difficulty in walking. Within 4 months, despite using deionized water for preparation of the dialysate, his condition progressed and his speech became markedly dysarthric, frequently unintelligible and occasionally, at the end of dialysis, he was mute. Comprehension and writing skills however were maintained. A further 2 months later he was readmitted to hospital following a series of grand mal convulsions and died shortly afterwards.

Questions

1. From what condition was this man suffering?
2. What preventative measures can be employed?

Comment

There are many neurological disorders that may be associated with renal disease or its treatment. They include manifestations of the primary disease such as mononeuropathy of diabetes or amyloidosis, hypertensive encephalopathy and cerebrovascular disease due to prolonged hypertension. In chronic renal failure, high serum levels of unidentified protein metabolites may be responsible for the peripheral neuropathy and also for a 'uraemic' encephalopathy consisting of asterexis, convulsions, insomnia and myoclonus. Similar transient disorders of brain function may be due to acute fluid and electrolyte imbalance. Treatment may result in neurological disorder such as steroid induced psychosis and convulsions, or in the disequilibrium syndrome, thought to be due to rapid fluid shifts between intra- and extracellular compartments in the brain engendered by a fast and efficient dialysis. Convulsions may also be precipitated by the too rapid infusion of hypertonic solutions, for example bicarbonate, which is particularly dangerous since it also partially neutralizes the protective effect of acidosis on hypocalcaemia.

This patient shows the typical features of a particularly distressing syndrome known as 'dialysis dementia' or 'dialysis encephalopathy'. This condition, which may in the past have affected up to six chronic haemodialysis patients in 1000 in Europe, is characterized by a slurring dysarthria and an apparent expressive dysphasia which may progress to mutism, and is most noticeable at the end of dialysis. It occurs in conjunction with disorders of movement and memory and with episodes of confusion and hallucination. Initially symptoms disappear between dialyses but later they become persistent. Abnormalities on the EEG may precede clinical features. Once the condition was recognized many epidemiological features became apparent: it was restricted to a few geographically defined areas and was far commoner in patients using an untreated domestic supply of soft water with which to make the dialysate; if deionized water was used or a process known as 'reversed osmosis' (which removes electrolytes) was incorporated into the dialysate delivery system the incidence was much lower. All this information suggested that it was due to an environmental agent found in the water used for dialysis and there is now much evidence to implicate aluminium as the toxic constituent. The role of oral aluminium compounds used as phosphate binders is not yet completely resolved.

Pathogenetically, a progressive uptake of aluminium by the body results in its deposition in the brain, more particularly the grey matter. Concomitant incorporation in bone results in 'fracturing osteodystrophy'. Current evidence suggests that oral aluminium is less important than that in the water supply as regards the development of the bone disease. It has also been suggested that aluminium may in part be responsible for the diminished erythropoiesis found in some patients. Originally, dialysis dementia was described as a severe, progressive disease and thought to be irreversible, with some patients dying within one year of its clinical onset. In some subjects it apparently progressed despite transplantation. It is now apparent that it should be preventable by the judicious use of deionizers and reverse osmosis. There are now some reports of reversibility by using desferrioxamine, a chelating agent which is given intravenously and acts to mobilize the aluminium. In the short term the serum levels rise, but this enables it to be dialysed out using dialysate fluid of very low aluminium concentration.

Case 39

Mr M. D.

A 19-year-old Asian textile spinner was referred for a second opinion. He was of short stature (150 cm) and weighed 41 kg, with knock knees. At the age of 5 he passed a number of renal stones, then he had no further trouble until one year ago when he developed right-sided abdominal pain, initially thought to be dyspeptic. However a plain abdominal x-ray showed bilateral nephrocalcinosis and on intravenous pyelography the right pelvicalyceal system which was only faintly outlined appeared distended. At operation a stone was removed from the right ureter but there was little improvement in the function of the right kidney. During this admission results showed sodium 145 mmol/ℓ, potassium 3.5 mmol/ℓ, urea 7 mmol/ℓ (42 mg/100 ml), chloride 107 mmol/ℓ, creatinine 110 μmol/ℓ (1.2 mg/100 ml), creatinine clearance 45 ml/minute, serum uric acid 0.4 mmol/ℓ (6.6 mg/100 ml), calcium 2.4 mmol/ℓ (9.7 mg/100 ml), phosphate 1.4 mmol/ℓ (4.5 mg/100 ml), alkaline phosphatase 95 IU/ℓ, serum albumin 40 g/ℓ with a total protein 80 g/ℓ. Astrup: pH 7.44, base excess 0. Twenty-four hour urinary calcium 5 mmol/ℓ (20 mg/100 ml) with 0.75 g of protein in a volume of 3 ℓ. An acid load test produced an astrup: pH 7.3, base excess −5 mmol with a minimal urinary pH of 5.8. X-rays of the lumbar spine showed multiple growth arrest lines. There was no evidence of tuberculosis.

Questions

1. What are the three possible diagnoses?
2. What further tests would you like to do?

Comment

The three conditions that can cause radio-opaque renal stones with evidence of distal tubular defects are (1) primary renal tubular acidosis, (2) medullary sponge kidney, and (3) primary hyperoxaluria. Normally an acid load test with oral ammonium chloride (0.1 g/kg) should result in a urinary pH of below 5.3 which this patient failed to achieve suggesting that he had a functional lesion of distal renal tubular acidosis. He also has high urine volumes possibly due to an impaired concentrating capacity, a common finding in patients with distal tubular acidosis.

The question arises as to whether the renal tubular acidosis is primary or secondary. The pattern of nephrocalcinosis may help. In primary renal tubular acidosis, medullary calcium deposits tend to be small and arranged in clusters corresponding to the pyramids of the medulla. In this case the deposits were like aggregates of small calculi in the smallest calyces implying that any impaired acidification and concentrated capacity is secondary. These appearances would be compatible with medullary sponge kidney (MSK) but the IVU failed to show the small evaginations from the calyces which are characteristic of MSK.

We are left then with primary hyperoxaluria producing radio-opaque calcium oxalate stones with secondary distal tubular defects. This diagnosis was confirmed by finding that the urinary oxalate was raised at 2 mmol/24 hours (180 mg) (normal is up to 0.32 mmol/24 hours (28 mg)).

Primary hyperoxaluria is a rare genetic abnormality transmitted as an autosomal recessive. It is undetectable in the heterozygote. Biochemically two different enzyme defects produce hyperoxaluria, although clinically they are indistinguishable. Most cases present in childhood and die in adolescence of renal failure, rarely patients live until middle age. Calcium oxalate crystals are deposited throughout the body in the kidneys, bone marrow, myocardium, testes, arterial walls and joint spaces occasionally giving rise to pseudogout.

There is controversy about treatment. In patients with good renal function pyridoxine and orthophosphates have been shown to reduce the rate of new stone formation. As renal failure occurs the urinary excretion of oxalate decreases. This results in rising serum levels and an accelerated deposition of oxalate crystals throughout the body. Because this is an incurable systemic disease haemodialysis is not offered in many centres. Transplantation is contraindicated; with early progressive failure of the graft. This is due to rapid deposition of oxalate from the previously accumulated large body pool.

Secondary hyperoxaluria which may cause renal stones, though not renal failure, is found in inflammatory bowel disease and after gut bypass operations. These patients have an increased intestinal absorption of oxalate and consequently hyperoxaluria. The urine however does not contain either glycolic or L glycenic acids which are present in the primary disease. Treatment in these patients is with cholestyramine. Other rarer cases of secondary hyperoxaluria are due to pyridoxine deficiency (a co-factor in the oxalates metabolic pathway), and high oxalate food ingestion, e.g. rhubarb.

The renal tubular acidosis in our patient was treated with Scholl's solution. However, over the next 7 years his renal function slowly declined and he eventually died of chronic renal failure at the age of 26.

Case 40

Mr S. Y.

One morning, Mr S. Y., a 64-year-old bus conductor, noted that the urine was frankly blood-stained throughout the stream. There were no other symptoms, in particular, no pain. Later the same day the urine was pink and by the evening was clear and remained so. However, he attended his family doctor and was referred to a Renal Clinic. There had been no urinary frequency, nocturia or dysuria. He had neither hesitancy or urinary dribbling. He had been well otherwise, and his weight was steady. He had worked in public transport all his life.

On examination he was not cachectic or clinically anaemic. Blood pressure was 150/85, heart normal, no heart failure. Neither kidney was palpable and the bladder could not be felt or percussed. The prostate was normal on rectal examination and the external genitalia showed no abnormalities.

Investigations: serum creatinine 105 μmol/ℓ, haemoglobin 13.5 g/dl, no proteinuria. Urine clear but haematuria on dipstick testing and 2 000 000 red blood cells/hour in a 2 hour timed urine. MSU was sterile.

Questions

1. What further investigations should be performed?
2. What is the probable diagnosis?
3. What is the therapy?

Comment

The urine deposit should be examined carefully. If there are casts or if, on phase contrast, the red cells appear distorted, this is suggestive evidence that the bleeding is glomerular. An IVU should be performed and a cystoscopy is mandatory.

In this patient the urine deposit showed no casts and well-formed red blood cells. The IVU showed normal kidneys and upper tracts but the bladder outline was irregular. Cystoscopy revealed extensive carcinoma.

The incidence of carcinoma of the bladder is second only to that of the prostate in malignancies of the urinary tract. Seventy-five per cent of the cases occur in males over the age of 50 and it constitutes 7% of all male carcinomata. Careful history taking may reveal an occupational association. This is important as there is the potential of an industrial injury claim. Some authorities suggest that this occurs in 20% of all cases of bladder carcinoma. There are carcinogens in materials used during curing rubber and in the dye industry, and it has been suggested that these may be present in agents used by tailors and perhaps hairdressers. Heavy cigarette smoking is statistically associated with carcinoma of the urinary bladder. Cyclophosphamide therapy for another malignancy can cause a chemical cystitis which may proceed to malignant transformation.

Treatment is by diathermy, by irradiation or by cystectomy. Such definitive surgery may be required even after an initial lesion has been treated apparently successfully by irradiation or diathermy since recurrence at a different area in the bladder is well recognized.

A single episode of painless haematuria, as in this man, is frequently associated with multiple papillomata in the bladder wall. These, although precancerous, are in themselves benign. When seen at cystoscopy, a biopsy is taken and the lesion(s) then treated by diathermy. In such cases repeated cystoscopy at 6 month intervals should always be performed to ensure that no further growths have developed.

In older men, painless haematuria may arise not only from kidney or bladder, but from congestion of the periurethral or prostatic vessels, as a benign, isolated incident.

Case 41

Miss R. T.

An 18-year-old shop assistant was found to have proteinuria early in her first pregnancy. In the last trimester hypertension and ankle oedema developed and an elective Caesarean section was performed at 36 weeks resulting in a live male infant weighing 2.45 kg. Postpartum, proteinuria persisted at 10–15 g/day, and she was referred for further investigation. No other family, personal or social history was found to be relevant. She had been taking frusemide and hydralazine as prescribed. Examination revealed three abnormalities: (a) gross oedema of the lower limbs up to thighs, (b) blood pressure of 155/110 mmHg supine and 150/100 mmHg erect, and (c) marked loss of subcutaneous fat of the face and upper limbs.

Questions

1. What name is applied to the condition described in (c) above?

2. What histological diagnosis might be confidently predicted?
3. What is the nature and effect of the abnormal circulating plasma component?

Comment

The characteristic anatomical findings described are those of partial lipodystrophy (PLD) which is frequently associated with type II mesangiocapillary glomerulonephritis (dense deposit disease or DDD) and C3 nephritic factor (C3 Ne F), a circulating immunoglobulin of the IgG class, that acts to stabilize the alternate pathway C3 convertase. This leads to C3 consumption with a low level of detectable C3 in serum and, therefore, a lack of total haemolytic complement (THC) activity as determined by red cell lysis. Production of C3 is also decreased.

Investigation of this patient confirmed heavy proteinuria with a lowered plasma albumin, plasma creatinine of 250 μmol/ℓ (2.8 mg/100 ml), and a calculated creatinine clearance of 21 ml/minute. This apparent impairment of renal function was at least in part 'pre-renal', in that hypoalbuminaemia predisposes to hypovolaemia. Her THC activity was less than 20% of normal and C3 measured at 15 mg% (normal being 100–200 mg%). C3 Ne F was present. Renal biopsy revealed a well established mesangiocapillary glomerulonephritis (MCGN) previously called membranoproliferative or chronic lobular proliferative glomerulonephritis, and electron micrographs demonstrated intramembranous electron-dense deposits. Immunofluorescence was strongly positive for C3 but negative for other complement factors and immunoglobulins.

Surprisingly, in view of her disease, and particularly the widespread crescent formation, proteinuria has diminished to 4g/day, plasma albumin risen to 37 g/ℓ and serum creatinine stabilized at around 120 μmol/ℓ (1.4 mg/100 ml) with a creatinine clearance of 45 ml/minute some 16 months since first assessment. Prognosis however must remain guarded.

Histologically MCGN shows an increase in mesangial cells and matrix and an increase in glomerular basement membrane (GBM) thickness, but it is not a homogeneous condition, subdivisions being based on the localization of electron-dense deposits and the appearance of the GBM. Formerly only two types were described but it is now common to recognize three. In all three, mesangial deposits can be detected. In Type I MCGN deposits are also located in the subendothelial area and the GBM remains intact, the increase in thickness being due to interposition of the mesangium between the GBM and the endothelial cell. This lesion can occur with 'shunt' nephritis or hepatitis B infection. Evidence, both serological and immunofluorescent, suggests that activation of the complement cascade is via the classical pathway and there is a tendency to find slightly depressed, or low normal, serum levels of the early components namely Clq, C4 and C2 with these same factors and immunoglobulins demonstrable in the glomeruli. Type III MCGN was previously classified with Type I but here deposits may also be subepithelial, and the GBM may be frayed. Furthermore, complement activation is probably via the alternate pathway.

In Type II MCGN, the deposits are found within the GBM. This lesion is frequently found in patients with PLD and C3 Ne F resulting in a profound lowering of circulating C3 but normal C2, Clq and C4. Usually C3 alone is demonstrated in the glomeruli without the other components or immunoglobulins. It is interesting to note that PLD, with or without C3 Ne F, may be found without clinical evidence of glomerular disease, and similarly, not all patients with Type II MCGN have PLD or C3 Ne F detectable. It is possible that C3 Ne F had once been present, since its disappearance from the serum is reported. Just as intriguing is the undoubted occurrence of PLD and C3 Ne F with Types I or III rather than Type II MCGN. Recurrence of Type II MCGN in a transplanted kidney is well recognized.

Typically, MCGN presents in childhood or adolescence, with any one of the glomerular syndromes. The outlook is held to be poor whatever the histopathological subgroup, with a cumulative mortality reaching 50% by 11 years from onset. One trial, reported recently, failed to show any long-term benefit from combination therapy with cyclophosphamide, warfarin and dipyridamole as compared to placebo. However, there is some evidence that high-dose alternate-day treatment with steroids for at least one year does prolong survival in children, particularly if therapy is started early, with Type I patients apparently doing better than Types II or III.

Case 42

Mrs S. B.

A 33-year-old lecturer had noticed increasing breathlessness for a month. For two weeks vision in the right eye had been blurred, and intermittently, she wakened with frontal headache and nausea. She had also experienced nocturia up to 3 times per night for at least 6 weeks. There had been no paroxysmal dyspnoea or angina. She had undergone right pyelolithotomy 10 years previously and a single parathyroid adenoma had been removed a year later.

On examination there were operation scars in the neck and right loin. Pulse 80/minute regular, blood pressure 240/150 mmHg. JVP not elevated, no oedema. Apex beat was forceful but localized and not displaced. A fourth heart sound was present but no murmurs; crepitations audible at the right base; neither kidney was palpable, no abdominal murmur. Fundi showed bilateral papilloedema, narrow irregular arterioles, haemorrhages and 'soft' exudates with the right perimacular area particularly involved. Investigations were: haemoglobin 11.4 g/dl, WCC $10.3 \times 10^9/\ell$ (70% polymorphs), platelets $200 \times 10^9/\ell$, ESR (Westergren) 45 mm/hour, plasma urea 30 mmol/ℓ (180 mg/100 ml), plasma creatinine 560 μmol/ℓ (6.3 mg/100 ml), plasma sodium 134 mmol/ℓ, plasma potassium 4.2 mmol/ℓ, plasma chloride 92 mmol/ℓ, plasma HCO_3 19 mmol/ℓ, plasma calcium 2.3 mmol/ℓ (9.2 mg/100 ml), plasma phosphate 1.2 mmol/ℓ, urinary calcium 3 mmol/day, urinary protein 1.5 g/day, creatinine clearance 15 ml/minute, ECG left ventricular 'strain' pattern, chest x-ray pulmonary oedema, IVU equal kidneys 12.5 cm in length, with bilateral nephrocalcinosis and a 'staghorn' right calculus, poor concentration of dye bilaterally.

Questions

1. What is the probable sequence of events leading to the presentation?
2. What further investigations may help?
3. What is the prognosis?

Comment

The findings suggest that accelerated hypertension has developed in the course of pre-existing renal disease. Before primary hyperparathyroidism was cured surgically, the plasma calcium was 3.5 mmol/ℓ (14 mg/100 ml). Radiology showed no evidence of osteoclasis on the phalanges, but there was nephrocalcinosis and renal stone formation with super-added infection. Blood pressure was 160/110 mmHg and creatinine clearance was reduced to 30 ml/minute.

Urinary infection persisted and was difficult to eradicate; new renal calculi formed and these changes contributed to progressive renal damage exacerbated by the eventually aggressive hypertension.

Parathyroid hormone increases calcium absorption by small bowel *and* renal tubule. However, there is hypercalcuria; the hypercalcaemia which results from accelerated bone resorption and increased calcium absorption from the gut raises the filtered load at the glomerulus beyond the increased tubular resorptive capacity so, renal damage has two components — from tubulointerstitial calcium deposition, related to the hypercalcaemia and increased calcium resorption and from renal stone formation, consequent on the hypercalcuria (*see* p. 142).

Tubulointerstitial calcium deposits are largely invisible on x-ray, producing at most the tiny parenchymal opacities of nephrocalcinosis. Nevertheless, the present case is an example of how the damage produced can be both severe and irreversible; renal biopsy in similar patients shows interstitial and intratubular calcium deposits, tubular atrophy and (secondary) glomerular loss as the damaged nephrons become ischaemic.

Accelerated hypertension complicates the course of about 5% of patients with chronic renal failure and has a 'vicious circle' effect, the extensive small vessel damage diminishing still further the GFR.

This patient required vigorous hypotensive therapy using vasodilators, diuretics and β-blockade, the last introduced cautiously because of the cardiac failure, but *not* contraindicated when this failure is the result of hypertension which may be controlled by such drugs.

Regular haemodialysis was required within a year. Mrs S. B. has now undergone a successful renal transplant operation.

Case 43

Mr A. L.

A 69-year-old retired post office engineer was referred by his GP for further investigation after finding a raised blood urea. He gave a 3 month history of vague ill health, anorexia and weight loss with a metallic taste in his mouth and had a dull aching pain in the loins and lower back. There had been no haematuria, dysuria or frequency. He had been treated with steroids for 5 years for biopsy proven temporal arteritis. On examination he was wasted, pulse rate 90 beats per minute regular and blood pressure 170/90 mmHg. No abdominal masses were found and no loin tenderness was elicited. Results: urea 12.6 mmol/ℓ (76 mg/100 ml), creatinine 240 µmol/ℓ (2.7 mg/100 ml), Hb 9.5 g/dl, MCV 80 fl, normochromic normocytic, WCC 7.3 × 10^9/ℓ with a normal differential. ESR 58 mm/hour. An MSU contained less than 1 pus cell and no red cells per high power field with no casts and no growth. A 24 hour urine contained 0.2 g of protein. An IVU showed a poorly functioning right kidney, the left side had a dilated pelvicalyceal system with dilatation along most of the length of the left ureter. Cystoscopy with easy retrograde ureteric catheterization demonstrated dilatation of both upper tracts, which were obstructed at the level of L_4—S_1. The ureters appeared to be pulled medially and had poor peristalsis. A diagnosis of retroperitoneal fibrosis was made and surgical ureterolysis performed (dissection of the ureters from their fibrous plaque). Biopsy of the tissue encasing the ureters showed interlacing bundles of fibroblasts and collagen, with no evidence of neoplasia.

Questions

1. What causative agents have been implicated?
2. What other organs may be affected?

Comment

Retroperitoneal fibrosis is an overgrowth of fibrous tissue in the lumbar region, rarely extending into the pelvis, causing obstruction to the ureters. The aetiology is uncertain although most cases are idiopathic as in this patient and occur in middle age in either sex. An immune process may be involved. In some subjects recurrent small haemorrhages from an atheromatous or aneurysmal aorta give rise to a fibrous reaction which encases the ureters. Methysergide, an antiserotonergic drug used to treat migraine has been associated frequently with retroperitoneal fibrosis. Methyldopa may have been involved in a few cases. Practolol which causes sclerosing lesions of the visceral peritoneum and small bowel does not affect the retroperitoneal tissues. Malignancy usually due to local spread of intra-abdominal tumours can give a very similar picture both on x-ray and at surgery.

There are no specific symptoms or signs in the presentation of retroperitoneal fibrosis. There is a combination of vague ill health, anorexia, weight loss, pyrexia and a high ESR sometimes associated with acute, subacute or chronic renal failure. Oedema of the legs may occur due to involvement of the inferior vena cava and a hydrocoele formed if the venous drainage of the testis is impaired. Fibrosis may be found at other sites, around the rectosigmoid, scrotum, heart valves, mediastinum and pleura. Pleural effusions are a rare form of presentation.

The disease can be unilateral, however, even when bilateral one side is often affected before the other as in this patient. An IVU and retrograde cystoscopy are the primary investigations for diagnosis though ultrasound, and CT scanning, and Hippuran renography will give similar information. Radiologically, there is either unilateral or bilateral hydronephrosis. The involved ureter is often kinked and pulled medially with a characteristic, smooth 'rats tail' tapering near the pelvic brim, ureteric peristalsis is absent. Confirmation of the diagnosis and exclusion of malignancy is by biopsy of the fibrous tissue.

Treatment is either medical or surgical. If methysergide is implicated this should be stopped immediately. Regression of fibrosis has been reported though some cases continue to progress. Oral steroids (prednisolone 60 mg/day) are occasionally beneficial in the idiopathic variety. Surgical intervention gives the best results with the ureter dissected and secured lateral to the fibrous plaque. Recovery of impaired renal function may occur if the damage is acute, though the disease may recur. Long-term prognosis is surprisingly good as it is often a self limiting disease.

In the patient described one year later urea was 10 mmol/ℓ (60 mg/100 ml), creatinine 190 μmol/ℓ (2.1 mg/100 ml) and Hb 13.5 g/dl.

Case 44

Mr D. S.

For many years this 43-year-old man had been a keen amateur runner and marathon participant. He now found training had become tiring and, over 3 weeks, he developed anorexia and noticed that his urinary stream was slower. There was also a scant yellowish penile discharge. Suddenly, he became very ill with rigors, severe perineal and low back discomfort and strangury and was admitted as an emergency. There was no earlier history of urinary symptoms. He denied extramarital sexual contact. On questioning his wife, she mentioned that she had recently noted a yellowish vaginal discharge. Salient features on examination were: temperature 40 °C, blood pressure 115/65 mmHg, suprapubic tenderness and exquisite tenderness over a distended left prostatic lobe on rectal examination. There was no epididymo-orchitis. Haemoglobin 13.0 g/dl, WCC $18.0 \times 10^9/\ell$ (90% polymorphs), MSU grew *E. coli* sensitive to gentamicin and Septrin. Blood cultures, sterile.

Questions

1. What is the diagnosis?
2. What other investigations should be performed?
3. What is the management?
4. What are the pathogenesis and prognosis of the underlying condition?

Comment

This man has an acute urinary tract infection, predominantly an acute prostatitis. There is a close relationship between bladder urine infection, prostatitis and posterior urethritis. Clinically, it is difficult to separate the three precisely. Prostatitis indicates that the prostatic acini and surrounding tissues are inflamed, particularly close to the urethra. Ascending infection via the urethra is thought to be the common path, the patient's own bowel flora being the usual site of the infecting organism. It has been postulated that *E. coli* may be transmitted to the urethra from the partner during intercourse.

Prostatitis may be

(a) acute or, as in this case, subacute; an aggressive bacterial infection causing severe systemic upset,

(b) relapsing; sometimes associated with a recurrent urinary infection, the same organism persisting in the prostatic fluid where, once chronicity is established, antibacterial agents are not rapidly effective. The symptoms are those of recurrent dysuria without much systemic upset,

(c) recurrent; the prostatic tissue being distorted, different organisms cause infection with perineal and urethral discomfort from time to time.

It is important to remember that prostatitis may follow gonococcal infection. In order to establish that there is prostatitis in the absence of acute prostatic symptoms, it is worthwhile collecting a three glass urine, that is obtaining the first few millilitres of urine, an ordinary MSU and then a specimen following firm prostatic massage. If there is prostatic infection a profuse discharge following prostatic massage or the presence of a very large number of pus cells in the postprostatic massage specimen are helpful in diagnosis.

Acute prostatitis may settle completely but during the episodes urethral obstruction commonly occurs and, in any case, it is always wise to check by IVU that there is no underlying abnormality of the urinary tract. This can best be done when the acute attack has subsided. It is important to treat with effective antibiotics for a prolonged period of time, a minimum course of 10 days is required and if symptoms have not completely subsided, this may be continued for at least one month. Post-treatment urine should always be examined and the prostate palpated rectally to ensure that it has returned to normal. Should chronic symptoms arise the choices are regular prostatic massage with a prolonged course of antibiotic therapy or, if this is ineffective and there is evidence of chronic urethral obstruction, transurethral prostatectomy may be valuable. The organisms responsible for prostatitis are usually *E.coli* or *Staphylococcus aureus*. However, mycoplasmata, chlamydia and trichomonas have also been incriminated.

Case 45

Mr J. O.

A 24-year-old Nigerian student of food technology was admitted as an emergency. He had been generally unwell for several weeks. On Christmas Eve one week previously he had presented to casualty with abdominal pain and constipation. He was tender over the descending colon and rectal examination revealed gross faecal residue but otherwise examination was normal. He was sent home with a laxative and glycerin suppositories. Following a 999 call he was brought back to casualty a week later complaining of abdominal pain with swelling of his abdomen and face, breathlessness and a low urine output. He had experienced no joint pains, rashes or sore throats. He had returned from Nigeria one month previously. He had had malaria 8 years previously.

On examination he was pyrexial at 38 °C and looked ill. He had leuconychia and there was gross oedema with anasarca and facial oedema. There was a left pleural effusion, ascites and synovial effusions in both knees. Jugular venous pressure was only detected on lying flat and blood pressure was 115/100 mmHg lying, 90/70 mmHg standing.

Results showed Na 131 mmol/ℓ, K 3.6 mmol/ℓ, calcium 1.83 mmol/ℓ (7.5 mg/100 ml), urea 15.9 mmol/ℓ (95 mg/100 ml), creatinine 300 μmol/ℓ (3.4 mg/100 ml), albumin 15 g/ℓ, total protein 44 g/ℓ, Hb 12.3 g/dl, WCC 5.4 × 10^9/ℓ, MCV 65, sickle test normal, Hb electrophoresis normal. Pleural fluid contained 0.6 g/ℓ protein. Ascitic fluid no growth. No TB seen. There was a non-selective urinary protein loss of up to 30 g/day. Serum amylase, SCAT, Latex, ANF, WR, ASOT and blood cultures were all normal or negative. MSU showed hyaline and granular casts. An IVU showed normal size kidneys. There was no evidence on ultrasound of renal vein thrombosis.

Questions

1. What is the immediate management?
2. What is the diagnosis?

Comment

This is a case of severe nephrotic syndrome which needs simultaneous symptomatic treatment and investigation. Treatment with high dose frusemide and spironolactone, salt restriction with a high protein and carbohydrate diet combined with albumin infusions resulted in clearing of the oedema and effusions and settling of the abdominal pain and temperature. Once the ascites had settled hepatosplenomegaly was found.

Abdominal pain is a well recognized feature of severe nephrotic syndrome and several patients have had unnecessary laparotomies because of it. The cause is thought to be either low serum amino acid levels or serum lipoprotein abnormalities secondary to the nephrotic state. Apart from this 'idiopathic' variety other causes of abdominal pain associated with nephrotic syndrome are renal vein thrombosis, peritonitis (without perforation) and pancreatitis.

In view of the history, malaria has to be excluded by thick blood films to look for parasites and if these are negative antibody titres may confirm a recent infection. A renal biopsy is also necessary to clarify the histology.

Raised antibody titres to *Plasmodium malariae* confirmed a recent infection though no parasites were found in the blood. Renal biopsy supported a diagnosis of malarial glomerulonephritis with variable segmental glomerular lesions with thickening and splitting of basement membranes. Immunofluorescence showed coarse granular deposits of IgM and IgG.

Malaria is said to be the most common cause of nephrotic syndrome in the world. It is also important because it was the first demonstration of a specific antigen associated glomerulonephritis in man. Using immunofluorescent antisera on renal biopsy tissue coarse granular deposits of IgM, IgG and C3 are found in the same distribution as malarial antigens. This suggests that the glomerulonephritis is due to the deposition of soluble antigen/antibody complexes in the glomeruli. Other parasitic agents implicated in immune complex glomerulonephritis are schistosomiasis and congenital toxoplasmosis. There is strong epidemiological evidence of a causal role for infection with *Plasmodium malariae*. The nephrotic syndrome is more common in areas where malaria is endemic and the frequency decreases with successful malarial eradication campaigns.

The natural history of malarial nephrotic syndrome is variable with poor prognosis found in cases with severe proliferative glomerular changes, persisting heavy proteinuria and raised malarial antibody titres.

Treatment with steroids has no benefit but long-term antimalarial prophylaxis is advised as relapse can occur with reinfection. Acute renal failure occurs rarely in malaria as part of the 'blackwater fever' syndrome of disseminated intravascular coagulation and haemoglobinuria precipitated by quinine treatment in a hyperinfected host.

Unfortunately our patient took his own discharge and returned to Nigeria believing his illness was due to a curse that could only be lifted by the local witch doctor.

Case 46

Mr B. D.

A 14-year-old boy was referred to his local hospital following an episode of frank haematuria. The only history available was of left loin pain of a few days' duration one week earlier, but with no associated infections and no history of renal colic or of passing a calculus. He denied any recent trauma, and no other relevant symptoms were forthcoming. Examination was entirely normal, and investigation revealed no abnormality in renal function or urinary tract anatomy as demonstrated by IVU and cystoscopy. Proteinuria was not present.

His subsequent follow-up was erratic and no further macroscopic haematuria was noticed, but infrequent testing of his urine always revealed microscopic haematuria. At the age of 16 years he came under our care and extensive investigation confirmed the presence of urinary red cells but 24 hour protein excretion was less than 1 g on four consecutive occasions. Creatinine clearance was 90 ml/minute. No other biochemical, haematological or immunological abnormality was detected. On reviewing the history it became apparent that his father had been investigated (IVU and cystoscopy) for an incidental finding of microscopic haematuria some years earlier. No abnormality had been detected and the matter had not been pursued. There was no other family history of renal disease. The paternal family of eight paternal siblings, paternal grandfather, 7 of 12 first cousins and our patient's own 3 siblings were, however, further investigated. Microscopic haematuria was confirmed in grandfather, father, uncle, and 2 siblings. Only in his elder sister was proteinuria in excess of 1 g demonstrated. All had normal renal function. None was deaf.

Our patient subsequently developed proteinuria in excess of 1 g and was subjected to renal biopsy.

Questions

1. What diagnoses might be entertained?
2. What other renal diseases may occur within families?

Comment

Any of the causes of haematuria (as outlined elsewhere) must of course be considered since, although unlikely, all these related people may have independent causes for blood in the urine. However, assuming a familial association, and that it is a constitutional trait rather than common exposure to an environmental insult, and in view of the apparent dominant mode of inheritance, Alport's syndrome or adult polycystic disease would feature in the differential diagnosis. The absence of deafness, although not an essential feature of hereditary nephritis, and the longevity of the possibly affected grandfather would militate against the former diagnosis. Normal IVUs in patient and father and the finding of normal renal function in all subjects including grandfather excludes polycystic disease.

Biopsy in our patient revealed mesangial proliferative glomerulonephropathy with immune complex deposition, and this latter feature again makes the diagnosis of hereditary (i.e. Alport type) nephritis unlikely. The immunofluorescent pattern was that of IgM and C3, IgG and IgA being absent, and therefore the diagnosis is not that of Berger's disease (IgA nephropathy). Mesangial proliferative glomerulonephritis, clinically manifest as benign recurrent haematuria, may be familial. Unfortunately we have been unable to examine biopsy material from other family members. Interestingly, we were able to show that no single HLA haplotype was shared by all the family members with haematuria.

Other glomerular diseases that may run in families includes the autosomal recessive Finnish type congenital nephrotic syndrome, which is invariably fatal in infancy.

In view of the association of Berger's disease, idiopathic membranous nephropathy and minimal change disease with certain HLA antigens it is surprising that other primary glomerular diseases are not more common in families than appears to be the case. We do have examples of familial clustering of cases but they are rare. Renal disease can also occur in association with inherited biochemical defects such as occur in gout, Fabry's disease, cystinuria and cystinosis, renal tubular acidosis and other even rarer conditions.

There is some evidence that ureterovesical reflux may be more common in children of individuals with such reflux. Finally, in any situation where the same disease occurs in family members, the possibility of exposure to a common environmental insult must be considered.

Case 47

Miss S. K.

A 15-year-old schoolgirl presented with a 1 year history of progressive weakness. She had difficulty in walking or lifting herself up. She complained of anorexia which had made the previous 6 months schooling barely tolerable.

She had always been thirsty — 'always at the tap' her mother said — and had lifelong nocturia and occasional enuresis. She was of small stature, a younger sister having outgrown her.

Because of the weakness, she was referred to a neurologist who found a predominantly proximal myopathy. Reflexes and sensation were normal. He considered a metabolic cause, and investigations showed blood urea to be 50 mmol/ℓ (300 mg/100 ml). She was referred to us for further management.

On examination, she was small (155 cm) and frail (39 kg), with pasty skin and pale mucosae. Blood pressure 90/60 mmHg lying, 70/50 mmHg standing, apex beat not displaced, 1/6 mitral murmur, no clinical abnormalities were found in chest or abdomen. She was myopic with nystagmus on lateral gaze. There was genu valgus, no localized muscle wasting but a proximal myopathy. She had a 'shuffling' gait.

Initial investigations showed Hb 6.5 g/dl, plasma urea 53 mmol/ℓ (318 mg/100 ml), plasma creatinine 600 μmol/ℓ (6.8 mg/100 ml), calcium 1.65 mmol/ℓ (6.6 mg/100 ml), phosphate 2.20 mmol/ℓ, alkaline phosphatase 225 IU/ℓ, creatinine clearance 3 ml/minute (uncorrected for surface area), proteinuria 2.5 g/day. IVU, skeletal survey, parathyroid hormone and vitamin D levels were obtained during the admission.

Initially, she received peritoneal dialysis, and with adequate resalination, her weight rose to 42 kg and blood pressure to 115/90 mmHg without a postural drop. She was given a 50 g protein diet with 50 mmol of salt daily and 1600 kcal, equivalent to 200 kcal/g nitrogen in the diet. Sodium chloride capsules were prescribed to maintain salt intake of 150 mmol/day. The plasma phosphate was reduced by dialysis and then controlled by aluminium hydroxide capsules. Then, 1-alpha hydroxycholecalciferol was prescribed. Thereafter, she maintained stable biochemistry with a GFR of 10 ml/minute and was much improved clinically.

Questions

1. What is the probable diagnosis?
2. What is the probable sequence of events leading to admission?
3. How should she be managed?

Comment

The long history of thirst and nocturia suggest that the renal disease was congenital or acquired at an early age. The family had not considered that these were features of a disease, rather that they were 'just her'. Uraemic symptoms (nausea and anorexia) were very recent on the other hand, so the primary lesion probably affected the renal medulla most prominently. This seems likely to be an example of medullary cystic disease, also termed 'nephron-ophthisis' in which small corticomedullary and intramedullary cysts occur, which do *not* lead to renal enlargement. Instead, with time the kidneys become shrunken and scarred. The most common genetic pattern is autosomal recessive. Polyuria, polydipsia and enuresis are features. Impaired urinary concentrating ability and sometimes renal sodium wasting are contributing factors. The slow progression of renal impairment and the eventual azotaemia developing in adolescence is reflected in pronounced metabolic bone disease and by hyperparathyroidism, features which are most evident in such circumstances.

The IVU showed rather small (9.5 cm) kidneys with irregular out-lines and poor dye excretion. The pelvicalyceal systems and bladder appeared normal.

Apart from mild 'knock-knee', the skeleton was normal on exami-nation. This suggests that, in early growth, skeletal metabolism was normal, further evidence that advanced uraemia was recent, influencing adolescent development. Radiologically, a skeletal survey showed indistinct bone texture generally, with increased density of the vertebral endplates ('rugger-jersey' spine), ill-defined metaphyses and widened epiphyses of the long bones (renal rickets) and, in the hands, subperiosteal erosions on the phalangeal margins (hyperparathyroidism). Bone age was 12 years, consistent with growth arrest during the development of the features of renal bone disease.

Serum 25 hydroxycholecalciferol ('vitamin D') level was 11 pg/ml (normal 10–25), yet 1:25 dihydroxycholecalciferol was not detected, indicating failure of 1-hydroxylation by the kidney and consequent unavailability of this potent dihydroxy metabolite of vitamin D, which promotes calcium absorption and possibly its incorporation into the bone front; neither of these essential ingredients of bone development is normal in advanced uraemia.

Hyperparathyroidism was confirmed, the plasma parathyroid hormone level was elevated 6–7 times above the normal range at 7.2, when plasma calcium was 2.0 mmol/ℓ (8 mg/100 ml). The high levels of parathyroid hormone in uraemia are the result of abnormal stimulation of the glands by the raised plasma phosphate level both directly and through its influence in lowering the plasma ionized calcium level by a mass action effect.

She eventually underwent subtotal parathyroidectomy with good effect. Bone healing occurred now under the influence of 1-alpha hydrocholecalciferol with oral calcium supplements.

Case 48

Mr E. R.

A 68-year-old man is admitted under the surgeons with abdominal pain. However, after 3 days of oliguria with a rising urea and creatinine a renal opinion is requested. He has a complicated history, initially presenting 15 years ago with an acute meningitic reaction to frontal sinusitis. X-rays taken at the time showed an enlarged pituitary fossa and he received a course of external x-ray therapy to his pituitary chromophobe adenoma. Six years ago he developed an iron deficiency anaemia secondary to a bleeding gastric ulcer and was treated with Caved-(S). and iron. At the time he had the typical features of pan-hypopituitarism and measurement of pituitary hormones confirmed the diagnosis. Treatment was commenced with thyroxine 0.15 mg daily, cortisone 12.5 mg daily and testosterone 250 mg i.m. once monthly. He remained well until the week before admission when he developed swelling of the ankles and shortness of breath, which did not respond to diuretics prescribed by his general practitioner. Three days prior to admission he had a severe abdominal pain and an episode of diarrhoea and vomiting, and he was unable to take his tablets. At the same time he developed a severe vasculitic rash on his legs. His urine output decreased and he was admitted to hospital in a semicomatose state with a diagnosis of an Addisonian crisis precipitated by either pancreatitis, gastroenteritis or a perforated ulcer. Blood pressure was 100/60 mmHg with a pulse of 60. He had a right pleural effusion and crepitations at the left base. His jugular venous pressure was raised 4 cm and there was bilateral ankle and sacral oedema. Abdominal examination showed generalized tenderness but no rebound or guarding. Investigation results showed Hb 10.6 g/dl, WCC $6.4 \times 10^9/\ell$, platelets $302 \times 10^9/\ell$, ESR 70 mm/hour, blood urea

33 mmol/ℓ (198 mg/100 ml), creatinine 440 µmol/ℓ (4.9 mg/100 ml), potassium 5.0 mmol/ℓ, calcium 1.9 mmol/ℓ (7.6 mg/100 ml), albumin 25 g/ℓ, amylase 140 IU/ℓ. Blood cultures and faeces were sterile. Coagulation tests were normal. An MSU showed hyaline casts and 100 RBC/high power field. ANF was positive for IgM and IgG although anti-DNA antibody test was negative. SCAT and Latex were strongly positive. There was no subdiaphragmatic gas on abdominal x-rays. On starting steroid replacement therapy his general condition improved but the rash persisted. He remained oliguric with fluid retention and required peritoneal dialysis before a renal biopsy could be performed.

Questions

1. Do you think he has acute tubular or glomerular damage?
2. Are there any more tests you would like to do to make the diagnosis?

Comment

This is a complicated case of a man with pan-hypopituitarism who presents with acute renal failure. A possible diagnosis is that he had an episode of gastroenteritis precipitating an Addisonian crisis because he was unable to take his steroid tablets. The ensuing hypotension owing to fluid loss and steroid depletion results in acute tubular necrosis. However, the history indicated that ankle oedema developed before his abdominal symptoms, suggesting that the renal problems came first. An important physical sign was the vasculitic rash on his legs. This together with the positive SCAT, Latex and ANF indicate an acute immunologically mediated injury. An urgent renal biopsy is therefore indicated. This showed pro-teinaecious deposits within capillary lumena and Bowman's space giving positive IgM and IgG immunofluorescence. Blood samples kept at 37 °C before separation of serum showed the presence of a monoclonal IgM Kappa cryoglobulin. Lymphocytic infiltration of the bone marrow together with the other findings would support the diagnosis of cryoglobulin associated glomerular damage.

Cryoglobulins are immunoglobulins which form precipitates, gels or crystals in the cold. The clinical features are caused by obstruction of small blood vessels particularly in the skin where the temperature is lower. Cryoglobulinaemia is classified into three types. Type I are monoclonal immunoglobulins usually IgM or G associated with either Waldenström's macroglobulinaemia or multiple myeloma and which precipitate when the concentration is high, resulting in a vasculitic purpuric rash or causing Raynaud's phenomenon. Type II is when a monoclonal protein, usually IgM is directed against the Fc portion of IgG. Cryoprecipitation occurs when immune complexes of IgG and IgM anti-IgG are formed. Patients present with widespread vasculitis, arthritis and glomerulonephritis. Type III is when there is polyclonal IgM cryo-globulin reacting with IgG. It is often associated with SLE, poly-arteritis nodosa or rheumatoid arthritis.

The case described is an example of Type II. There was no evidence of a lymphoma, myeloma or Waldenström's macro-globulinaemia. He was treated with pulse steroid therapy (1 g Solu-Medrone/day for 5 days), then prednisolone 100 mg reducing to 10 mg over 3 weeks and adding chlorambucil 10 mg daily. His renal function recovered and the vasculitis disappeared.

In summary this is a case of IgM monoclonal cryoglobulinaemia in a patient with pan-hypopituitarism and possible gastroenteritis.

Case 49

Mr H. F.

A 52-year-old golf club steward was referred to the Rheumatology Clinic with a 6 month history of pain, morning stiffness and swelling of his joints, notably wrists and knees. Examination revealed a rheumatoid nodule of the right elbow, tenosynovitis of the flexor tendon of the right thumb, swollen tender wrists, wasted quadriceps muscles and subluxed metatarsophalangeal joints. Serological investigations, originally negative for rheumatoid factor, sub-sequently became positive, and treatment was started with aspirin. Urinalysis was negative for albumin and glucose; haemoglobin 13.5 g/dl, ESR 50 mm/hour. Because of progressive erosive arthropathy he was commenced on gold therapy. Following a test dose of sodium aurothiomalate 10 mg, he received a further 50 mg i.m. weekly for 2 months. Regular urinalysis was negative for albumin until the eighth week. Gold therapy was immediately withdrawn. The proteinuria persisted and he developed a frank nephrotic syndrome with proteinuria in excess of 10 g/24 hours, dependent oedema and a serum albumin of 26 mg/ℓ. Other investigations heically mediated is supported not only by the time course of symptoms and positive immunofluorescent findings, but like the idiopathic form of membranous nephropathy it develops more commonly in individuals who are HLA DRW3 positive.

A disparate group of other drugs have been implicated in the pathogenesis of immunologically mediated glomerular disease, including the anticonvulsant troxidone, and the anticoagulant phenindione as well as tolbutamide, phenylbutazone and bismuth, mercury and lithium containing compounds: membranous nephropathy is the most frequently identified lesion but proliferative, focal and minimal changes are also reported. The glomerulotoxicity of the angiotensin converting enzyme inhibitor captopril and the chelating agent penicillamine, however, may be related to the possession of sulphhydryl groups. Proteinuria is reported in about 1% and 7% respectively of patients receiving these drugs.

Case 50

Mr K. H.

Six years ago a 42-year-old police superintendent was referred for investigations by his GP. Six weeks prior to the clinic appointment he had had an episode of port wine coloured urine followed by left renal colic. A day after this he passed some 'sludge' in his urine. Four days later he had a second similar episode. When seen in clinic he was asymptomatic, and fit looking with no abnormal physical findings on examination. Investigations done at that time showed a normal MSU with < 1 RBC or WBC per high powered field and no casts. No organisms were seen. Hb was 15.4 g/dl, WCC $4.9 \times 10^9/\ell$, urea 6.0 mmol/ℓ (30 mg/100 ml), creatinine 90 μmol/ℓ (1.0 mg/100 ml). An IVU showed no abnormality in the kidneys or urinary tract and a chest x-ray was normal. He was placed on the waiting list for cystoscopy but was lost to follow-up for two years because of an administrative error. He was re-referred having had three more episodes of port wine coloured urine. One of these was painless but two were associated with left loin pain. Examination was normal with no abdominal masses felt. An MSU taken at this time showed 100+ RBC per high powered field. Urea was 7.0 mmol/ℓ (42 mg/100 ml), creatinine 95 μmol/ℓ (1.1 mg/100 ml), Hb 14.0 g/dl, WCC $6.0 \times 10^9/\ell$, ESR 95 mm/hour. An urgent IVU in comparison to the one two years previously showed an increase in the size of the lower pole of the left kidney with distortion of the lower calyceal system.

Questions

1. What further investigations need to be done?
2. What is the diagnosis?
3. What is the prognosis?

Comment

The initial history was suggestive of renal colic but investigations were normal. The case is of haematuria, loin pain, high ESR and a space occupying lesion in the kidney.

An ultrasound scan should be performed to show if the renal lesion is cystic or solid. If it is solid the most likely diagnosis is of a clear cell carcinoma of the kidney — a hypernephroma. Angiography has a confirmatory role in order to delineate the lesion and demonstrate its pathological blood supply.

Hypernephroma is the most common renal carcinoma, classically presenting with haematuria, flank pain and a palpable mass. Pyrexia of unknown origin can be caused by a hypernephroma as can nephrotic syndrome due to renal vein thrombosis caused by obstruction of the renal veins by the tumour growing into them. 'Ectopic' hormone production may give rise to polycythaemia secondary to erythropoietin, hypertension due to renin or hypercalcaemia due to a parathyroid like substance. Amyloid and a peripheral neuropathy are rarer occurrences. Secondary spread is blood borne, to lung, liver, bone or brain due to embolization of tumour cells from the local spread into the renal veins. 'Cannon ball' metastases on chest x-ray are typical in the lung. Following nephrectomy there may be regression of these secondaries though if possible local metastases should be resected.

A very high ESR is occasionally found as in this case. Often the patients have no symptoms until the tumour is very large when the abdominal mass can be misdiagnosed as spleen or liver on palpation.

Treatment by radical nephrectomy can lead to cure though the overall 5 year survival rate is approximately 30%. In this patient nephrectomy was performed, although the patient had a further episode of haematuria 2 years later. Investigation showed a second hypernephroma in his remaining kidney. He had the remaining kidney removed and has been well on dialysis for over a year with no evidence of recurrence. Successful treatment of hypernephroma in a solitary kidney by subtotal nephrectomy has been reported.

Case 51

Mr L. M.

A 58-year-old dustbinman was admitted to hospital having had an epileptiform seizure. He had been perfectly well until 3 months previously when he had first attended his general practitioner because of progressive tiredness and lethargy. More recently he had complained of increasing bilateral deafness and blurring of vision. Two weeks before admission he had attended a local casualty department with epistaxis. He had had purulent sputum for the previous two days.

On admission he was confused, drowsy and incoherent. Temperature was 38 °C and there were coarse crepitations at the left base. Blood pressure was 160/80 mmHg lying, 150/60 mmHg sitting. Fundi showed bilateral retinal haemorrhages and venous engorgement.

Results: Hb 10.0 g/dl normochromic normocytic, WCC 12.1 × $10^9/\ell$, platelets 150 × $10^9/\ell$, ESR 95 mm/h, urea 15 mmol/ℓ (90 mg/100 ml), creatinine 150 µmol/ℓ (1.7 mg/100 ml), Ca 2.5 mmol/ℓ (10 mg/100 ml). Arterial pH 7.3, PCO$_2$ 35 mmHg, PO$_2$ 90 mmHg. Coagulation studies normal.

Questions

1. What further tests would you like to do?
2. What is the diagnosis?
3. What is the treatment?

Comment

The symptoms are of hyperviscosity syndrome and chest infection with dehydration. The plasma viscosity in this patient was grossly elevated at 7.56 centipoises (normal 1.5 centipoises). The two main diseases that cause a hyperviscosity syndrome are myeloma and Waldenström's macroglobulinaemia. The latter is characterized by a high serum content of monoclonal IgM in the serum, enlargement of the lymph nodes, bleeding (possibly due to a factor X deficiency) and anaemia. The peripheral blood may show a lymphocytosis and the bone marrow be infiltrated by lymphocytes which are producing the abnormal paraprotein. The skeleton is not affected in this disease, with no lytic lesions.

The diagnosis of myelomatosis depends on two of the following three factors — a paraprotein in serum or urine, atypical plasma cells in the marrow and lytic skeletal lesions.

Waldenström's macroglobulinaemia accounts for the vast majority of cases of hyperviscosity syndrome although this is being recognized increasingly in myeloma. The size of the abnormal protein molecule as well as its plasma concentration contribute to the pathogenesis of hyperviscosity. Aggregations of monoclonal paraprotein molecules to form large molecular weight complexes so producing hyperviscosity is particularly common in the rare sub-class of IgG_3 and also with IgA. In patients with IgG myeloma the paraprotein concentration is always greater than 50 glℓ and frequently greater than 100 g/ℓ when symptoms of hyperviscosity are present.

Measuring the plasma viscosity is only a guide. Symptoms may be present with only slightly elevated values while some patients may be asymptomatic at high levels.

In the case described there was an IgG Kappa paraprotein with total protein 98 g/ℓ and albumin 21 g/ℓ. A bone marrow showed 30% atypical plasma cells and multiple lytic lesions were present in the skull and pelvis. The diagnosis is therefore an IgG Kappa myeloma. The patient was rehydrated with intravenous normal saline and given antibiotics but he still remained confused with a persisting plasma viscosity of 6.5 centipoises. Plasmaphoresis was then performed with a dramatic improvement in his general condition. Within 12 hours he became completely rational and mentally alert. Chemotherapy was commenced for his underlying myeloma with good results.

Case 52

Mrs M. F.

A 50-year-old lecturer had been maintained for over 10 years on 2 g daily of lithium carbonate which satisfactorily controlled her manic depressive illness. For 4 months she had noticed thirst, polydipsia and polyuria. On direct questioning she admitted to a gain of 20 kg in weight over the previous 3 years but no other symptoms. She was obese, 106 kg in weight with a blood pressure of 120/80 mmHg and no retinopathy, neuropathy or proteinuria. The serum lithium concentration was, at 0.7 mmol/ℓ, within the therapeutic range. Random fasting and 2 hour postprandial blood sugar levels were 28, 24.2 and 33.8 mmol/ℓ (504, 436 and 608 mg/100 ml) respectively. Glucose intolerance is not a recognized feature of lithium therapy and in the absence of ketonuria a diagnosis of maturity onset diabetes mellitus was made.

With institution of a low carbohydrate diet her weight decreased, urine became sugar free and random blood sugar levels fell to the normal range, but polyuria persisted and progressed reaching in excess of 9 ℓ/day.

Questions

1. How would you confirm the presumptive diagnosis?
2. What treatment is available and what precautions need to be employed?

Comment

Polyuria is a feature of: diabetes mellitus (which had been adequately treated in this patient); hypokalaemia and hypercalcaemia (which were excluded by the appropriate biochemical investigations); psychogenic polydipsia and diabetes insipidus (DI). Central DI may be due to impaired or absent antidiuretic hormone (ADH) production as a consequence of neurohypophyseal disease, e.g. tumour or trauma, or may occur as an idiopathic, sometimes familial disease. Nephrogenic DI occurs when the kidney is unable to respond to ADH or its analogues; it may be an X-linked recessive tubular defect affecting young males or may be induced by damage to the distal nephron by disease (e.g. Bence–Jones proteinuria) or drugs (e.g. lithium).

The diagnosis of nephrogenic DI due to lithium toxicity was made in this patient after demonstrating an inability to decrease her urine flow following water deprivation and an inability to increase the urine osmolality, despite a 3% fall in body weight. Following administration of desmopressin (dDAVP) there was still no substantive response. The differential diagnosis from psychogenic polydipsia is more difficult since prolonged polydipsia may impair both ADH release and renal responsiveness, but as the history was of an acute onset and there was no diurnal variation in symptoms, compulsive water drinking was not thought likely. Acquired nephrogenic DI is said however to rarely result in 24 hour urine volumes greater than 5 ℓ . An important diagnostic point is the finding that a patient with psychogenic polydipsia has normal responses following water deprivation, or vasopressin administration without water deprivation, in that they achieve relatively greater urine concentration with the former manoeuvre. The converse is found in genuine diabetes insipidus.

Central or 'true' DI may be alleviated by using nasal sprays of vasopressin (short acting) dDAVP (medium acting) or with intramuscular injections of vasopressin in oil (long acting). Chlorpropamide may help symptoms in some patients. In both central and nephrogenic DI, thiazide diuretics may act to decrease urine flow substantially. The mechanism for this paradoxical effect is uncertain.

In our patient it was felt unwise to discontinue the lithium therapy which was controlling her psychosis so well, and she was started on bendrofluazide. This had the expected effect of causing a rise in serum lithium due to increased resorption and initially her daily dose of lithium had to be reduced. With time, the daily requirement frequently reverts to the original dose. Her urine output fell rapidly to 5.5 ℓ /24 hours.

Between 10 and 30% of patients on a therapeutically effective dose of lithium are reported to develop vasopressin resistant polyuria. Lithium is the best known drug possessing this capability but it can also occur with the tetracycline demeclocycline (which can be used in the treatment of inappropriate ADH syndrome where water restriction is ineffective) and following the use of the anaesthetic agent methoxyfluorane. Both renal tubular acidosis and acute renal failure are reported in association with lithium therapy, and goitrous hypothyroidism is a well recognized complication of prolonged administration.

In cases of severe acute intoxication dialysis may be used to remove the drug.

Case 53

Mr S. J.

A 45-year-old unemployed steel fixer began vomiting and was admitted under the surgeons. He was referred as a case of acute renal failure when his biochemical results were available. His history went back 18 months when he had developed peritonitis secondary to a perforated diverticulum and an emergency, defunctioning, transverse colostomy was performed. He recovered slowly after a stormy course and 6 months later an elective sigmoid resection was carried out with end-to-end anastomosis, the colostomy being closed. At this time his results were Na 135 mmol/ℓ, urea 4.2 mmol/ℓ (25 mg/100 ml), creatinine 90 μmolℓ mg/100 ml), Hb 14.5 g/dl.

He remained well until 6 days prior to this admission when he developed hiccoughs, vomiting and heartburn. He had been unable to keep down any solid food, although he had been drinking water. There had been no abdominal pain and no haematemesis or melaena. His urine volume had decreased over the previous 3 days.

On examination he was alert, orientated and apyrexial. Over the pectoral area skin turgor was decreased. Pulse was 100 regular with blood pressure 120/80 mmHg lying and 110/60 mmHg sitting. Heart sounds were normal and there was no oedema. On neurological examination Chovstek's and Trousseau's signs were positive. There was an epigastric succession splash. Results showed Hb 17.3 g/dl, WCC $14 \times 10^9/\ell$, PCV 0.538, Na 111 mmol/ℓ, K 5.6 mmol/ℓ, Cl 85 mmol/ℓ, urea 58 mmol/ℓ (348 mg/100 ml), creatinine 250 μmol/ℓ (2.8 mg/100 ml), Ca 2.4 mmol/ℓ (9.8 mg/100 ml), amylase 420 IU, blood sugar 4.4 mmol/ℓ (79 mg/100 ml), serum osmolality 294 mmol/kg, arterial astrup pH 7.52, $P\mathrm{CO_2}$ 34 mmHg, $P\mathrm{O_2}$ 98 mmHg, actual bicarbonate 25 mmol/ℓ, urine Na 4 mmol/ℓ, urea 400 mmol/ℓ. X-rays showed a large gas bubble in the stomach. An MSU showed no white blood cells, less than 5 red blood cells and no casts per high powered field.

Questions

1. What is the diagnosis?
2. What is the management?

Comment

This is a case of hyponatraemia with uraemia and hypochloraemic metabolic alkalosis. Clinically there is evidence of fluid depletion from the decreased skin turgor and postural hypotension. The positive Trousseau's and Chovstek's signs are due to the alkalosis which has resulted in a fall in the plasma ionized calcium level even though the total serum calcium is normal. The low urine sodium is consistent with the low serum sodium and reflects a tubular conservation of intravascular salt and water. The urinary urea is high and appropriate to that in the serum. These findings show that the kidney has normal concentrating ability. Why then is the urea high and sodium low?

The serum sodium measurement is a concentration in extracellular fluid (ECF). A low value is a result of either a deficit in sodium in a normal ECF volume or a normal amount of sodium in an increased ECF volume or a combination of the two.

From the history vomiting is the major problem. Vomit contains sodium chloride approximately 75–150 mmol/ℓ together with a large number of hydrogen ions from the acidic stomach. The patient, to replace his fluid loss, was drinking water containing little sodium chloride or hydrogen ions. The salt and water lost has been partially replaced by water alone, this imbalance contributes to the hyponatraemia. There is also an element of volume depletion because the total fluid replacement is inadequate and has resulted in the postural hypotension, low skin turgor and uraemia. The metabolic alkalosis is produced by loss of hydrogen ions not by an excess of bicarbonate ions.

The situation described is rare and reflects high intestinal obstruction usually at the level of the duodenum. Frequently vomit contains bicarbonate ions from the duodenum so 'cancelling out' the effect of gastric juice hydrogen ion loss. However, in pyloric hypertrophy in infants, duodenal ulceration with scarring or perforation, or vomiting, as in this patient, hyponatraemia can occur.

Note particularly that the hyponatraemia only became apparent because of the replacement of lost salt and water by water alone.

In our patient adhesions from the previous peritonitis and surgery resulted in the duodenal obstruction. Treatment was by nasogastric aspiration and, most important, replacement of intravascular volume by normal saline. Within 2 days of fluid replacement urea was 3.0 mmol/ℓ (18 mg/100 ml) and creatinine 60 μmol/ℓ (0.7 mg/100 ml). The obstruction was then corrected surgically. The kidneys were *not* damaged and functioned promptly to correct the metabolic insult once sufficient fluids were provided.

Case 54

Miss D. B.

Miss D. B. a 22-year-old typist, having had no urinary symptoms in early life, now complained that over the past 3 years there had been 6 episodes of painful micturition with urinary frequency and suprapubic ache. Two years ago she had consulted her family doctor and on that and two subsequent occasions, antibiotics had been prescribed. No urine culture had been performed. A recent episode had been particularly painful and resulted in her attending the Renal Clinic. There had been no unexplained fever or abdominal pain in childhood, enuresis had not persisted after 3 years of age and at no time was there urinary hesitancy or dribbling. Her present symptoms had been exacerbated, and sometimes precipitated, by sexual intercourse. On direct questioning there were no symptoms suggestive of lumbar disc prolapse which could have caused impaired sacral nerve function.

On examination she looked well. Blood pressure 115/70 mmHg, there were no abdominal masses and no tenderness; neither kidney palpable. Vaginal examination: no discharge, healthy uterine cervix. There was no neuromuscular or skeletal abnormality.

Questions

1. What investigations should be performed?
2. What is the diagnostic category?
3. What advice should be given?

Comment

Practice varies in such cases. If symptoms are present a urine culture should be obtained. If there are no symptoms at the time of presentation, an early morning urine sample, obtained by the 'clean catch' method during the intermenstrual 14 days, should be examined microscopically and cultured. In the absence of symptoms such specimens may be repeated weekly for up to 6 weeks. If all these specimens are without deposit and sterile, the urine should only be cultured again when symptoms occur, and *before* antibiotic therapy is considered.

In Miss D. B., as in many such young women, none of the specimens obtained, when she was asymptomatic or while symptoms were present, contained bacteria of a single species at a concentration of at least 10^5/ml and so did not meet the Kass criteria for urinary tract infection.

The value of IVU is debatable. By far the majority of such cases have *no* renal upper urinary tract pathology. While cystoscopy rarely yields evidence of bladder inflammation, the urethral dilatation required may itself help to alleviate the symptoms. Urethroscopy prior to cystoscopy may show evidence of florid enlargement of the periurethral glands of Skene around the bladder neck.

The problems posed by dysuria and urinary frequency in young adult women have been extensively studied without definite conclusion. Only 50% of such presentations are associated with urinary tract infection as defined by Kass (see above). A further 30% have bacteria in the urine sample but not always of a single species. Even when Kass' criteria are met symptoms may be absent at the time, may persist even when the urine becomes sterile without antibiotic therapy or resolve even if a further urine specimen continues to show infection. Indeed, repeat urine specimens after a week become sterile in more than 50% of cases, without any antibiotic therapy.

It follows that the symptoms are not directly related to urinary tract infection as defined by Kass. Debate has continued as to the reason for these symptoms. A probable cause in many cases is local urethral trauma often exacerbated by intercourse. In some, but not all of such cases, periurethral gland inflammation may contribute and here urethral dilatation and sometimes fulguration of the glands may be helpful. Where there is distortion of the urethra, it is obviously more likely that organisms will become established in the periurethral tissues and so may lead to the minor bacterial counts frequently seen in patients complaining of the urethral syndrome. It is clear that, from time to time, there may be retrograde spread of these bacteria to the bladder and true urinary tract infection. However, the symptoms should be dealt with separately by reassurance, instruction regarding vaginal lubrication prior to intercourse and the exclusion of uterine cervical pathology or discharge since either of the latter may produce dysuria in its own right.

Antibiotics are rarely, if ever, required in this syndrome. Only if repeated specimens show a persisting urinary infection should they be offered and never without prior urinary culture. Indeed, repeated use of antibiotics in these cases may lead to further symptoms due to vaginal candidiasis.

The urethral syndrome can only be defined, of course, if there is no evidence of upper tract disease and plasma biochemistry is normal and there is no proteinuria or casts in the urine deposit.

Case 55

Mr M. B.

A 19-year-old garage mechanic was involved in a road traffic accident while driving his motorbike. The only injuries he sustained were an undisplaced isolated fracture of his pelvis and a penetrating wound of his left knee joint. There was no clinical suggestion of trauma to his kidneys or lower urinary tract, and he continued to pass urine normally. Routine urinalysis when admitted to hospital was unremarkable. Treatment consisted of surgical toilet to the left leg, intramuscular penicillin and tetanus toxoid and bed rest.

Within 3 days, the left knee joint became swollen, painful and inflamed and the patient was febrile. Pus was aspirated from the knee which grew a penicillin resistant *Staphylococcus pyogenes* and parenteral methicillin therapy was commenced. The response to treatment was rapid but, after a further few days, he developed a diffuse erythematous skin rash, the fever recurred and he became oliguric. Serum creatinine, which had been 90 μmol/ℓ on admission, had risen to 320 μmol/ℓ. A nephrological opinion was sought.

No further relevant history was elicited from this patient and physical examination, apart from some superficial abrasions and the skin rash, was uninformative except to demonstrate that there was no obvious fluid depletion. Examination of his fluid balance and blood pressure charts were similarly unremarkable. The urine contained blood and protein but no myoglobin. Serum potassium was 4.9 mmol/ℓ, full blood count showed an eosinophilia of 10% of a total WBC count of 12.8 × 10^9/ℓ. High dose intravenous urography demonstrated a faint bilateral nephrogram with normal sized kidneys, with no evidence of urinary tract obstruction.

Questions

1. What is the most likely diagnosis?
2. How should the patient be managed?

Comment

The presumptive diagnosis of a methicillin-induced interstitial nephritis was made and the offending drug withdrawn. A renal biopsy the following day confirmed the clinical diagnosis, showing a marked interstitial infiltration of lymphocytes, plasma cells and eosinophils and some evidence of tubular damage. Glomeruli were normal. The oliguria persisted for another 72 hours, during which time the skin rash faded and the patient was managed satisfactorily by fluid restriction and prophylactic oral administration of calcium resonium. His renal function recovered completely.

Drugs can affect renal function in a variety of ways, many of which remain subclinical. Some of the more serious manifestations are dealt with in other sections in this book. The drugs most frequently associated with an acute interstitial nephritis are antimicrobials such as ampicillin, methicillin, sulphonamides and rifampicin and some diuretics have also been implicated. This condition is relatively rare in clinical practice but is important to recognize since stopping the drug usually results in complete recovery. The pathogenesis is mediated via a hypersensitivity reaction, evidence of which is supported by the frequent association with rash, fever, arthralgia and peripheral blood eosinophilia. This has led to the occasional use of steroids in treatment but there is no satisfactory evidence that such intervention is superior to simply discontinuing the drug.

Some reports stress the finding of circulating antitubular basement membrane (anti TBM) antibodies and IgG and C3 deposition in the tubules.

Interstitial infiltrate may also occur in many other situations including an acute rejection episode in a renal transplant, chronic pyelonephritis and many patients with apparently primary glomerular disorders have significant interstitial abnormalities.

Case 56

Miss S. O.

In 1973 a 19-year-old geography undergraduate presented to the University Health Centre because of swelling of her ankles of a few days' duration. She had also been aware of a firm but painless swelling in her neck of a few weeks' duration but had not sought a medical opinion. Apart from an appendicectomy at the age of 11 years, and the 'usual childhood illnesses' her previous history was without incident, and her parents and two elder siblings were well. She had no symptoms suggestive of local disease to account for the swelling in her neck. Physical examination confirmed the presence of 'rubbery' lymphadenopathy in the left cervical region but no other nodes were felt in the gland fields and liver and spleen were not palpable. There was pitting oedema to mid calf but no other abnormal clinical signs. Heavy proteinuria was confirmed by dipstick testing.

In the course of the next few weeks she had a lymph node biopsy, staging laparotomy with splenectomy and a renal biopsy and was treated with radiotherapy alone for stage II Hodgkin's disease. (Chest radiographs had confirmed the presence of mediastinal lymphadenopathy.) With prompt remission of the lymphoma, the nephrotic syndrome also resolved.

She has remained well with no recurrence of disease for nearly 10 years.

Questions

1. How may malignant diseases affect the kidneys?
2. What histological appearance would be expected on the renal biopsy?

Comment

The effects of primary renal neoplasms are dealt with elsewhere in this book, however, non-renal malignancies may have a variety of nephrological consequences. The kidneys are relatively common sites for metastatic spread and infiltration, and this is particularly so with the leukaemias and lymphomas, although such secondary invasion is only rarely a cause of terminal renal failure. Metastases and primary tumours infiltrating around the lower urinary tract, e.g. carcinoma prostate or carcinoma of the uterine cervix, may be responsible for an obstructive uropathy.

Undesirable hormone production, such as inappropriate ADH secretion or ectopic production of a parathormone-like substance from a bronchial carcinoma may also affect renal function and myeloma and paraproteinaemia may have various effects on kidney structure and function as described in other cases in this book. Chemotherapeutic treatment of malignancies, particularly haematological ones, may cause acute renal failure due to hyperuricaemia and subsequent crystal precipitation in the tubules and collecting ducts. This can be avoided by the concurrent administration of allopurinol.

The patient described here, exhibits the interesting phenomenon of non-metastatic neoplasia-associated glomerular disease, of which there have been a number of reports over the last few years. One of the most frequent examples is of a membranous nephropathy developing in association with a carcinoma, usually of the lung but also of breast, skin, gut and other organs. Some authors have noted an incidence in excess of 10% of patients with membranous glomerulonephropathy having an underlying malignancy. The pathogenesis in such cases is thought to involve tumour, or tumour related products acting as the antigen in the production of immune complexes which are finally deposited in the glomerular basement membrane. In a few patients such antigens, and/or tumour specific antibodies have been eluted from renal biopsy tissue.

The other common association, as in this patient, is a minimal change lesion with normal optical microscopy, negative immuno-fluorescent findings but the usual foot process fusion demonstrated by electron microscopy, and Hodgkin's disease, the two usually developing concurrently, with the latter most often of the 'mixed cellularity' type histologically. The pathogenesis of the glomerular lesion, like that of otherwise idiopathic minimal change nephro-pathy, does not appear to be immune complex mediated and remains unexplained. This association however has been used to implicate a disorder of T lymphocytes in the genesis of such a lesion. Interestingly it is the common experience that with successful treat-ment of the malignancy, the glomerular lesion resolves; and with relapse, it may return.

Not all patients with glomerulopathy and carcinoma have membranous lesions and other histopathologies are reported. While a minimal change lesion is the most frequent association with Hodgkin's disease, membranous and proliferative lesions are described.

Other reported associations include the development of a Henoch–Schönlein syndrome with nephritis in patients with squamous cell carcinoma of bronchus and non Hodgkin's lymphoma, as well as the nephrotic syndrome occurring in subjects with chronic lymphatic leukaemia, many of whom appear to have a mesangiocapillary lesion.

This patient demonstrates clearly that an apparently primary renal disease may have underlying pathology, early diagnosis and treatment of which may influence the final outcome.

Case 57

Miss T. J.

A 15-year-old schoolgirl developed a discrete purpuric rash over trunk, arms and legs. There had been no previous relevant symptoms or other signs. Within one week she experienced tender, painful swelling of her ankles, knees, elbows and wrists in conjunction with intermittent abdominal pain. There was no nausea, vomiting or melaena. Urinalysis was unremarkable and her symptoms and signs subsided. A fortnight later the rash and arthralgia recurred and was soon followed by periorbital and ankle oedema. Following the discovery of blood and albumin in the urine she was admitted to hospital. No other positive features were elicited from the history; the only abnormalities on examination were the petechial rash predominantly over her legs, and pitting oedema of the lower extremities. Investigations: Hb 12.3 g/dl; platelets 259 × 10^9/ℓ; serum creatinine 80 µmol/ℓ (0.9 mg/100 ml); serum urea 5 mmol/ℓ (30 mg/100 ml); plasma albumin 21 g/ℓ; SLE cells, ANF, anti-ds DNA antibody levels, ASOT, IVU, SCAT and Latex tests all normal. Serum cholesterol 9 mmol/ℓ; 24 hour urine protein, 10 g; urine contained numerous red and some white cells (she was not menstruating and there was no growth on urine culture); serum immunoglobulin levels revealed a decreased IgG (4.5 g/ℓ), normal IgA (3.2 g/ℓ) and raised IgM (3.6 g/ℓ) with no monoclonal peak on electrophoresis.

Question

1. What is the diagnosis?

Comment

This young lady exemplifies the Henoch–Schönlein syndrome (HSS). There is no pathognomonic feature or diagnostic test, but the development of a rash, usually on the extensor surfaces of the lower extremities which may be originally urticarial but is later petechial, in combination with arthralgia of large joints (frank arthritis is less common) and colicky abdominal pain (in up to 50% of patients) which can be associated with small bowel petechiae or even intussusception, is quite typical. Bloody diarrhoea is a documented but infrequent accompaniment.

HSS is usually a disease of children less than 15 years of age with up to 50% being under 5 years old. Most series report an approximate ratio of 2:1, boys to girls, but with equal numbers of males to females in adult subjects. Various agents such as exposure to cold, β haemolytic streptococcal infection and drug reactions have been implicated in the aetiology. The clinical features are possibly the result of a common process which is triggered by a range of factors. HSS is an immune complex mediated disease (ICD); antigen/antibody complexes are found both in the circulation and at target organ sites, and antibody of the IgA class can be demonstrated even in apparently normal areas of skin of affected individuals. Spontaneous resolution of signs and symptoms generally ensues although a relapsing course is not infrequent. The development of renal disease is an important feature, but since the true incidence of HSS is unknown the frequency of renal involvement is impossible to determine accurately. It is estimated that from 10 to 50% of subjects are affected. Patients with recurrent HSS however have an increased likelihood of developing urinary abnormalities. Reports that glomerular disease is more common in adults almost certainly reflects bias in referral practice. The patterns of renal disease however are accurately described. There may be microscopic or macroscopic haematuria, (with or without proteinuria), a full nephrotic syndrome (with or without functional renal impairment) or even an acute nephritic picture with oligoanuria and hypertension. Histology too may be varied, with normal glomeruli on optical microscopy (although with immune complexes demonstrable under the electron microscope), or, the more common histological finding of focal proliferative change with IgA as the major localizing immunoglobulin and which is found predominantly in the mesangium. There is some evidence that glomerular histopathology may be present even if urinalysis and microscopy are normal.

Both diffuse proliferation and extensive crescent formation occur and these two groups have the worst prognosis with some patients progressing to terminal renal failure, most frequently within the first 1–2 years of the disease although there may be full clinical recovery. In general however, HSS with nephritis is a benign condition. We have observed patients with urinary abnormalities over prolonged periods of time. Most eventually remit, but occasionally there is a progressive decline in renal function. The effect of treatment with steroids and/or immunosuppressive drugs on the renal lesion is uncertain, but individual responses are reported.

An important point, is the possible late development of hypertension in patients with persistent, or intermittent urinary abnormalities. Careful follow-up, including for a period of time after all clinical activity appears to have resolved should be undertaken.

Complement may be involved in the pathogenesis of the renal lesion as certain complement components are found in the glomeruli on immunofluorescence. Variably depressed levels of circulating components can also be demonstrated. Such evidence can be interpreted to indicate that the alternate pathway of activation is predominantly involved.

We have seen patients with carcinoma bronchus and non-Hodgkin's lymphoma manifest a condition similar to that of HSS with renal involvement.

There are similarities between the nephritis of HSS and Berger's disease. The frequency of haematuria, the occasional finding of a raised serum IgA level, predominance of IgA on glomerular immunofluorescence as well as the generally uncommon progression to renal failure and even recurrence of disease following transplantation are all evidence of a relationship, as yet undefined, between these conditions. The biopsy in our patient revealed mesangial proliferation with focal and segmental accentuation. IgA and C3 were the predominant immunoglobulin and complement component on immunofluorescence, distributed in the mesangia and the basement membranes in a diffuse global and granular fashion. She was treated with loop diuretics and a high protein, low salt diet.

The proteinuria decreased over an 18 month period. At no time was she hypertensive or did renal functional impairment develop. Two and a half years from onset she was well and in full clinical remission.

Case 58

Mrs P. B.

A 32-year-old warden of flats for the elderly had complained for 3 years of intermittent right loin pain sometimes associated with passing dark red urine. Episodes occurred up to four times a year and lasted for 2 to 7 days. She had passed no calculi, there was no fever, dysuria or nocturia and no systemic illness. She had a daughter born 11 years ago after an uneventful pregnancy. One year ago she had a hysterectomy for menorrhagia. She denied regular analgesic intake. There was no previous medical or psychiatric history and no relevant family history.

On examination the mucosae were well coloured, tongue and nails normal and there were no petechaie. Blood pressure 135/80 mmHg. The right loin was tender on bimanual examination, but no abdominal organ or mass was palpable.

Investigation results showed Hb 15.0 g/dl, platelets $290 \times 10^9/\ell$, ESR 5 mm/hour, no evidence of a coagulation factor abnormality, serum creatinine 60 μmol/ℓ (0.7 mg/100 ml), potassium 4.5 mmol/ℓ, calcium 2.44 mmol/ℓ, urate 0.34 mmol/ℓ, creatinine clearance 107 ml/minute, no significant proteinuria, calcium excretion 4.0 mmol/24 hours, MSU 30 RBCs and less than 5 WBCs per high powered field, sterile, 2 hour timed urine 900 000 red cells/hour, no casts seen. Cystoscopy performed when there was no overt bleeding revealed no abnormality, IVU was normal. Renal angiography showed left kidney normal, right kidney showed ischaemic, probably infarcted, areas in the cortex with narrowed outer cortical vessels and dilated cyst like vascular abnormalities. Renal biopsy showed many dilated venules with no infarcted area in the specimen, occasional arterioles contained complement (C3).

Questions

1. What is the diagnosis?
2. What is the prognosis?
3. How should the patient be managed?

Comment

In the past 10 years patients have been described with a history similar to that of Mrs P. B. in whom selective renal arteriography is said to reveal narrowed cortical arterioles with areas of ischaemia. These areas on renal biopsy, are infarcted, the walls of adjacent arterioles containing complement (C3). This syndrome is virtually confined to young adult women and may be aggravated by oestrogen-containing oral contraceptives. Some evidence has been obtained of hormone associated alterations in platelet aggregation and the coagulation cascade in these patients.

However, the hypothesis that the loin pain haematuria syndrome is a pathogenic entity, the result of repeated renal cortical microinfarction in predisposed subjects, has not been accepted widely. The esoteric changes described by radiography, histopathology and haematological investigations have not been easy to reproduce. Furthermore, in many patients with loin pain and haematuria there are unusual personality traits with exaggerated suppressed anxiety and sometimes occult organic psychosis. Sometimes the claim that haematuria occurs and presentation with a urine sample containing blood, has been matched by the near simultaneous observation at cystoscopy that the bladder urine is free of red cells.

In our patient, unusual vascular anomalies occurred which are not typical of findings in other reports but point to an underlying, presumably congenital vascular anomaly.

Management was by periodic admission for bed rest and short-term analgesia. Some patients become dependent on analgesics and this must be discouraged. Extensive trials of agents to prevent platelet aggregation (aspirin, dipyridamole) have not been rewarding. Oral contraception with oestrogen preparations is best avoided.

The prognosis of this syndrome depends on its cause. There is no suggestion that, in idiopathic or other cases, progressive renal impairment occurs. Few patients present when aged over 40 and the symptoms appear to lessen with time, even when no cause has been determined. A combined approach by hospital and general practice may reveal occult analgesic abuse leading to renal papillary necrosis, or covert psychosis with fabrication of the haematuria.

It is worth remembering that small vascular anomalies in the pelviureteric system may bleed intermittently and are difficult to detect. The Osler–Rendu–Weber syndrome should always be considered, particularly if there is a family history of bleeding, if petechial lesions are present, or if unilateral symptoms are associated at cystoscopy with blood issuing from one ureter only.

2 Topics

Topic 1: Examination of urine

This involves the quantitative estimation of urinary constituents such as sodium, potassium, urea, creatinine, protein, calcium, cystine and uric acid; semiquantitative methods, most frequently using commercially available dipsticks, and detection and examination of formed elements in urine by microscopy. The quantitative measurements are the province of the clinical biochemist and will not be mentioned further in any detail.

Urinalysis

'Routine urinalysis' usually consists of dipstick testing. It is important to follow the instructions supplied with these reagents, specifically in keeping the sticks dry and in observing the colour changes at the correct time interval after immersion and withdrawal.

1. Protein is detected by its ability to alter the colour of indicators such as tetrabromphenol. The local pH is kept constant by incorporation of buffers in the test strip, and the indicator changes from yellow to green to blue depending on the amount of protein present in the urine. Two points are worth noting: (a) this is a sensitive method and as little as 150 mg/ℓ of protein may give a '+' result, (b) it does not detect Bence-Jones protein, which may however precipitate on heating and redissolve on further heating.
   More quantitative techniques for measuring protein in urine include salicylsulphonic acid, biuret and turbidometric methods.
2. Glucose. The test strip for detection of glucose is quite specific. It contains glucose oxidase, which, in the presence of glucose generates gluconic acid and peroxide. The latter, in the presence of peroxidase which is also impregnated in the strip, causes the other component, orthotolidine, to change from yellow to blue.
   'Clinitest' tablets, consisting of copper sulphate, citrate, sodium hydroxide and sodium carbonate when added to 5 drops of urine mixed with 10 drops of water causes the tablet to dissolve with the production of a hot alkaline solution. In the presence of reducing

substances, of which glucose is only one, the colour changes from blue to orange in a reasonably quantitative manner, due to the production of cuprous ions from cupric ions.
3. Blood. In this test, the strip contains peroxide and orthotolidine. In the presence of haem, which acts like peroxidase, oxidation of orthotolidine results in the change of colour to blue.

Urine microscopy

The enthusiasm for urine microscopy seems to vary from clinician to clinician and whether this is due to ability to interpret or to the value put on the findings is difficult to determine. Certainly some points are worth noting, namely the best results will come from a practised observer who is involved directly with the patient, and secondly that fresh urine should be examined. The novice should learn from an experienced teacher or make use of one of the handbooks or atlases of urine microscopy.

It is usual to examine unspun urine when urinary tract infection is suspected and the finding of large numbers of white cells and bacteria, in urine which has been collected properly (midstream), strongly supports the diagnosis although urine culture and colony count are still mandatory. Pyuria may be found in the absence of bacteriuria in such conditions as renal TB, calculus disease, glomerular disease, analgesic nephropathy and partially treated UTI. Bacteriuria without pyuria may also occur, particularly if urine is left before examination such that the few bacteria present multiply. The mean generation time for *E. coli* for example may be as little as 20 minutes, although in freshly voided urine left on the shelf at room temperature it is probably nearer one hour.

The value of accurate cell counts using a counting chamber as against a semiquantitative method (cells per high power field) is still disputed. Generally, the formed elements are concentrated by centrifuging 10 ml of urine for 5 minutes at 2000–3000 rpm. Ninety-five per cent of the supernatant is decanted and the sediment resuspended in the remaining 0.5 ml of urine. This is examined first with the low power and then the high power objective and the result recorded as cells/casts per high power field (hpf). Elements that may be expected are listed as follows:

1. Red blood cells (RBC): normal RBC excretion rates have been recorded at $1–2 \times 10^6$/24 hours. This approximates to 2 cells/mm^3 of unspun urine or a maximum of 1 cell per hpf. Up to 10 cells per

hpf have been recorded in the absence of detectable urinary tract disease. Increased excretion is found in association with fever and exercise. In pathological states, macroscopic haematuria may occur with infection, trauma, tumour or calculi anywhere from kidney to urethra. It may also be found with polycystic disease and some forms of glomerular disease. It has recently been shown that RBC of normal size and shape in urine originate from the collecting system, whereas abnormally shaped cells may indicate glomerular pathology.

2. White blood cells (WBC): normal WBC excretion rates are slightly higher than for RBC: $1-4 \times 10^6$ cells/24 hours, less than 5 cells/mm^3 of unspun urine or 1–2 WBC per hpf. Similarly exercise and fever may cause an increase in these rates. The situations where greater than normal WBC counts are found have been outlined above. Specific staining techniques may be indicated, in which case the finding of a high eosinophil count in urine may suggest an interstitial nephritis. Plasma cells are also noted in a few patients with myeloma.

3. Squamous epithelial cells: these large irregular shaped cells originating from ureter, bladder and urethra are a normal finding.

4. Renal tubular epithelial (RTE) cells: can be differentiated from WBC by their greater size ($\times 3$) and circular eccentric nucleus. They are only occasionally found in normal urine. Large numbers are indicative of tubular damage and in an appropriate clinical setting, support of the diagnosis of APN.

5. Casts are produced in the tubules and assume the shape of that tubule, i.e. cylindrical. The different types of casts have different diagnostic implications.

    (a) Hyaline casts are formed by the agglutination of Tamm Horsfall Glycoprotein (THG) which takes place in the tubules. They occasionally occur in normal subjects but are also present in a wide variety of renal diseases and increase during exercise and with fever. The precipitation of THG is increased in the presence of albumin and therefore such casts are a frequent finding in the urine of nephrotic subjects.

    (b) Granular casts are hyaline casts with added serum proteins such as albumin, gamma globulin or lipoprotein. The occasional cast is probably of the same significance as a hyaline cast but the presence of large numbers is indicative of underlying pathology, such as amyloid, diabetic, hypertensive or idiopathic glomerular disease or ATN.

(c) Cellular casts are important because they indicate that the cells originated in the renal parenchyma, and have become attached to a hyaline/granular cast. Red cell casts are of particular importance since they imply glomerular (or occasionally tubular) disease. White cell casts are found in acute pyelonephritis or interstitial nephritis.

6. Other formed elements may be found in the urine. Crystals of uric acid or oxalate are generally not indicative of specific pathology. Characteristically cystine crystals are seen in patients with cystinuria. Oval fat bodies, which are thought to be the catabolized lipoproteins leaking from the glomerulus and turned into cholesterol esters are lipid laden RTE cells. They are common in subjects with heavy proteinuria but require special stains or polarized light to be fully appreciated. Malignant cells may be detected but require special staining techniques and the interpretive skill of the experienced cytologist.

Topic 2: Creatinine clearance (Ccr)

Glomerular filtration rate (GFR) is that volume of plasma which is filtered across the glomeruli per unit time, and in the UK is usually expressed as millilitres per minute. It gives an index of renal function which is proportional to the number of intact nephrons. When the value obtained is corrected for height and weight (usually standardized to a surface area of 1.73 m^2), sex and age of the individual, it can be used to identify subjects with normal or impaired renal function, and to monitor progression or resolution of renal disease.

The measurement of GFR is based on the concept of 'clearance'. A substance present in plasma and urine is deemed to be 'cleared' from the body at a measurable rate, which is dependent on glomerular transmembrane pressure, (the difference between hydrostatic pressure in the capillaries and the oncotic pressure of the plasma) and the permeability and surface area (i.e. total number of glomeruli) of the membrane. The clearance (C) of a substance is then expressed as $C = \frac{UV}{P}$

where U = urine concentration of the substance
V = volume of urine produced/unit time
P = plasma concentration of the substance.

The clearance of any substance can then be measured, but in order to determine the GFR, such a substance must (a) be freely filtered across the glomerulus, (b) not be secreted or resorbed in the tubules or distal urinary spaces, and (c) be present at a constant level in the plasma. The biologically inert substance which fulfils criteria (a) and (b) is inulin and C_{inulin} is taken as the value for GFR. However there are problems in using this substance. It is not endogenous and therefore has to be infused i.v. until criterion (c) is fulfilled, or given subcutaneously. Furthermore, accurate collection of urine may necessitate bladder catheterization and since measurement of inulin concentrations is not a standard laboratory procedure, inulin clearance methods are not readily available in most hospitals.

Therefore use is made of creatinine, an endogenous product of muscle creatine phosphate breakdown. This is fairly constant and therefore criterion (c) is achieved. Creatinine is small enough to be freely filtered across the glomerulus, but is however secreted by the renal tubule. Except when GFR is severely impaired and tubular secretion rises giving a falsely high estimate of GFR, this potential error can be ignored.

In summary then,

$$GFR = C_{inulin} \simeq C_{cr} = \frac{U_{cr}V}{P_{cr}}$$

The major sources of error are

(a) overestimation of GFR when renal function is severely impaired, as outlined above,
(b) accuracy in the timed collection of urine. This is minimized by asking patients to collect 24 hour urine samples, and they must be instructed clearly how this is to be done. Twenty-four hour collection also eliminates error due to any diurnal variation in creatinine excretion.

Of course patient cooperation is essential. We have a patient who undoubtedly collects only his overnight urine in the bottle and tries to persuade us that this is a full 24 hour collection by adding tap water until what he considers to be the desired volume is present in the receptacle!

In the neonate values for GFR are approximately 50% of those achieved at one year (standardized to 1.73 m^2). From one year onward corrected values remain constant at about 110–130 ml/minute until about 30–40 years of age, after which they decline, reaching about 50% of maximum values at 60 years of age and 30% at

80 years. Interestingly, plasma creatinine values, in the absence of renal disease remain reasonably constant. This is because production rate diminishes, due at least in part to a decline in lean muscle mass.

Some authorities claim that provided GFR has been determined on one occasion, then if allowance is made for changes in weight, and age, renal function can be monitored at least as accurately, by serial plasma creatinine measurements alone. In ideal circumstances with a stable plasma urea and urine flow in excess of 2 ml/minute, urea clearance is approximately 60% of GFR. However, unless creatinine measurements are unavailable, there is no justification now for determining urea clearances. The variation in plasma levels and in tubular secretion rates, which are influenced considerably by urine flow, make these estimates inaccurate.

It is salutary to recall the different 'flow rates' concerning the kidney: renal blood flow is 1000 to 1200 ml/minute and therefore renal plasma flow approximates to 500 ml/minute; and with 20% filtration gives a GFR of 100 (to 130) ml/minute while urine flow is usually around 1 ± 0.5 ml/minute.

Finally, because of the ease of measurement, radioisotopes, particularly ^{51}Cr EDTA, have been used to estimate GFR.

Topic 3: Drugs in renal disease

The use of drugs in patients with renal failure can give rise to severe problems. Major modifications of dosage or complete avoidance may be necessary. Many drugs are metabolized by the kidney or excreted unchanged in the urine. Failure to excrete a drug or its metabolites may produce toxicity to the kidney or other organs (e.g. gentamicin), increased sensitivity (e.g. digoxin) or loss of effect when renal function is reduced (e.g. frusemide).

For several drugs with minor, non dose-related side effects, little modification in dosage is necessary. Where the efficiency and toxicity are closely related (a low therapeutic index) the recommended dosage schedules should be adjusted according to measured blood levels (e.g. gentamicin). The loading dose should be the same as the initial dose for patients with normal renal function. Subsequently alterations can be made either in the frequency or size of dosage or both.

Renal function declines with age and many elderly patients have a glomerular filtration rate less than 50 ml/minute while still having a serum creatinine in the normal range and dosage should be adjusted accordingly.

The following tables illustrate common drugs that are either nephrotoxic, need dosage adjustment of should be avoided in renal failure. If in doubt always check with the relevant literature.

Nephrotoxic drugs

Antibiotics	Damage	Comment
Aminoglycosides e.g. Gentamicin Streptomycin Amikacin Kanamycin Tobramycin Netilmicin	Also ototoxic	Monitor blood levels. Nephrotoxicity increased with concomitant dosage of frusemide.
Cephalosporins Cephaloridine Cephalothin	Proximal tubular damage	Avoid
Antifungal Amphotericin B	Distal tubular damage	Use only if no alternative
Antiarthritic Gold Penicillamine	Nephrotic syndrome Nephrotic syndrome	
Analgesics Phenacetin ? Paracetamol	Analgesic nephropathy	Avoid
Organic solvents Carbon tetrachloride	Proximal tubular damage + hepatic damage	Used in suicide attempts
Ethylene glycol (antifreeze)	Obstructive renal failure due to calcium oxalate in tubules	
Cis-platinum	Tubular damage	
Cyclosporin A	Tubular damage	Reversible

136

Drugs requiring dosage adjustment

Name	Complication
Infection	
Penicillin	Rashes more common
Ampicillin	
Carbenicillin	Neurotoxic, high sodium content
Benzylpenicillin	Neurotoxic, may produce fits
Cephalsporins	
Cefamandole	
Cefoxitin	
Cefuroxime	All possibly nephrotoxic
Cephazolin	
Cephradine	
Cephalexin	
Cotrimoxazole	Rashes and blood dyscrasias
Chloramphenicol	Depression of haemopoesis
Isoniazid	Peripheral neuropathy
Ethambutol	Optic nerve damage
Metronidazole	Neuropathy
Cardiovascular	
Digitalis	Arrhythmias
Disopyramide	Arrhythmias
Methyl dopa	Postural hypotension
Propranolol	Raised blood concentrations may reduce renal
Atenolol	plasma flow and decrease renal function
Metoprolol	
Frusemide } may require	Ototoxicity, rashes
Bumetanide } higher dosage	
Immunosuppression and chemotherapy	
Azathioprine	
Bleomycin	
Cyclophosphamide	
Melphalan	
Mercaptopurine	Increased marrow suppression
Procarbazine	
Thioguanine	
Methotrexate	

Drugs requiring dosage adjustment *(continued)*

Name	*Complication*
Gastrointestinal	
Cimetidine	Confusion
Metoclopromide	Extrapyramidal signs
Central nervous system	
Phenobarbitone	
Amylobarbitone	Slowly eliminated, accumulates
Anti-inflammatory + Analgesics	
Aspirin	
Indomethacin	
Brufen + other propionic acid derivatives	Fluid retention plus deterioration in renal function
Pethidine	CNS depression

Drugs to avoid if creatinine clearance < 20 ml/minute

Name	*Complication*
Metformin	
Phenformin	Lactic acidosis
Chlorpropamide	Hypoglycaemia
Talampicillin	accumulates
Cephaloridine	
Cephalothin	
Chloramphenicol	
Nalidixic acid	Rashes photosensitivity
Nitrofurantoin	Neuropathy
Tetracyclines	Antianabolic Increased urea. Use doxycycline.
Neomycin	Ototoxic, nephrotoxic
Ethacrynic acid	Ototoxic
Amiloride	
Triamterene	Hyperkalaemia
Spironolactone	
Carbenoxolone	Fluid retention
Methotrexate	Marrow suppression
Gold	Nephrotoxic
Penicillamine	Nephrotoxic
Probenecid	Toxicity increased
Pancuronium	
Tubocurarine	Prolonged paralysis

Topic 4: Renal tubular acidosis — the acid load test

Classic distal renal tubular acidosis (Type I) is characterized by a systemic acidosis with alkaline, or only weakly acid, urine. It may be familial or occur as part of an autoimmune disease (e.g. in association with Sjögren's syndrome or lupoid hepatitis) especially in young women.

Weakness due to hypokalaemia is a common presentation and nephrocalcinosis is often present. Diagnosis is established by finding a systemic acidosis with an alkaline urine or, if there is no acidosis, by undertaking an acid load test in which ammonium chloride provides sufficient hydrogen ions to induce a systemic acidosis. An abnormal test is when the urine pH does not fall below 5.3 and urinary titratable acid and ammonia excretion is low.

The rarer proximal tubular acidosis (Type II) is often associated with other proximal tubular defects (amino aciduria, renal glycosuria, hyperphosphaturia, hypouricaemia). The systemic acidosis is due to urinary bicarbonate wasting. However in contrast to the Type I disorder, if the plasma bicarbonate is below the proximal tubular threshold for bicarbonate the urine may be acid. If bicarbonate is infused until the plasma bicarbonate and pH are normal, bicarbonate passing into the renal tubules is not reabsorbed and so produces an alkaline urine. Bicarbonate infusion is not a routine test procedure and will not be dealt with in detail. The 'acid load test' is described below.

Acid load test

Equipment needed:

(a) Six 20 ml Universal glass bottles, numbered 1 to 6.
(b) Liquid paraffin.
(c) Measuring cylinder.

Procedure:

No fasting or water restriction necessary.

1. Patient has capillary Astrup taken before the test.
2. Urine specimen No. 1 taken. Volume recorded on bottle and time. If the urine volume is less than amount to fill bottle, liquid paraffin is used to cover top of urine, this prevents oxidation which raises the pH.

3. Ammonium chloride. 0.1 g/kg (acid load) is given. Patient instructed to take capsules slowly over half an hour. (It may make the patient nauseated.)
4. Urine specimen to be collected as in (2) at hourly intervals, or when patient can pass urine. The timing of each specimen is noted.
5. Approximately 4 hours after the start of the test patient has a further capillary astrup to check that he has developed a systemic acidosis.
6. Test finishes with the last urine sample approximately 6 hours after the ammonium chloride.

Topic 5: Water deprivation/vasopressin test

Water deprivation is used in conjunction with the administration of vasopressin to differentiate between central (neurohypophyseal) and nephrogenic diabetes insipidus. In the former there is diminished or absent ADH and in the latter, impaired renal tubular response to adequate ADH secretion.

No previous preparation is required, but on the day of the test the subject is denied access to fluid from 9.00 am until 5.00 pm. The test is stopped if more than 3% body weight is lost. Urine volume, and serum and urine osmolalities are measured hourly. At 5.00 pm i.m. vasopressin tannate in oil (10 units) is given and the patient allowed to drink. The same urine and serum measurements are continued.

A normal person will maintain serum osmolality between 280–295 mmol/kg, so that once fluid intake is restricted the urine osmolality will rise, and urine flow rates will decrease. In diabetes insipidus, urine production will continue unabated, urine osmolality will remain low and serum osmolality will start to rise.

Following the administration of vasopressin, the subject with central DI will show a decrease in urine output and a rise in urine osmolality. No such effect will be noticed in nephrogenic DI.

It is more difficult to establish a diagnosis of psychogenic polydipsia. However, providing the subject can be prevented from gaining access to water during the test, the urine osmolality should rise during water deprivation to a greater degree than following vasopressin administration. Psychogenic polydipsia can also be distinguished from central DI by infusion of hypertonic saline. Serum osmolality rises and there is a normal accompanying rise in serum ADH, which of course does not occur in central DI.

Topic 6: The chest x-ray in renal disease

Diagnosis	Case presentation
Hyperparathyroidism	42, 47
Tuberculosis	19
Hypernephroma	50
Pleural effusion	12
Hypertension	3
Wegener's granulomatosis	36
Multiple myeloma	5, 30

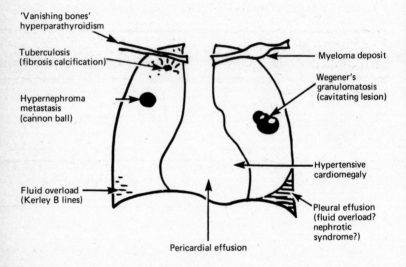

'Vanishing bones' hyperparathyroidism

Tuberculosis (fibrosis calcification)

Hypernephroma metastasis (cannon ball)

Fluid overload (Kerley B lines)

Myeloma deposit

Wegener's granulomatosis (cavitating lesion)

Hypertensive cardiomegaly

Pleural effusion (fluid overload? nephrotic syndrome?)

Pericardial effusion

The chest x-ray is the most frequently requested radiological investigation, and it may often show manifestation of diseases primarily distant from the chest, renal disease being no exception. A chest x-ray should be regarded as a routine investigation in all patients presenting with renal failure to assess fluid and cardiac state and to look for evidence of such diseases as Wegener's granulomatosis or multiple myeloma.

Topic 7: IVU interpretation and renal calcification

The IVU is the standard investigation to define both renal anatomy and, to a lesser extent, function. It is important to obtain good quality films. Sufficient contrast media should be used when there is poor renal function and tomography if renal outlines are obscured.

Interpretation of intravenous urograms

Diagnosis	Case presentation
Chronic pyelonephritis	31
Chronic glomerulonephritis	4
Polycystic kidney	2
Space occupying lesion	50
Papillary necrosis	15
Megaureter and hydronephrosis	1
Amyloid	30 + 20
Medullary sponge kidney	34
Tuberculosis	19

Cupped calyx   Cortex   Reduced cortex

Cortical scar

Medulla

Clubbed calyx

Normal calyx

NORMAL KIDNEY

CHRONIC PYELONEPHRITIS

CHRONIC GLOMERULONEPHRITIS

No loss of cortex

Stretched calyx

SOL

FETAL LOBULATION

POLYCYSTIC KIDNEY

SPACE OCCUPYING LESION (SOL)

Ring shadows

PAPILLARY NECROSIS

PELVI URETERIC JUNCTION (PUJ) OBSTRUCTION

MEGA URETER AND HYDRONEPHROSIS

Calcification

Distorted calyx

Streaks of contrast media

Calcification   Scarring

LARGE SWOLLEN KIDNEY

MEDULLARY SPONGE KIDNEY

RENAL TUBERCULOSIS

Amyloid   No calyceal deformity

Calcification in the kidney

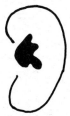 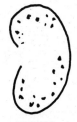 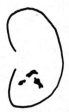

STAGHORN	DIFFUSE CORTICAL	DIFFUSE MEDULLARY	ISOLATED MEDULLARY
Reflux with infection	Old cortical necrosis (very rare)	Renal tubular acidosis (Type I) Hyperparathyroidism Pyelonephritis Sarcoid (rare) Primary hyperoxaluria Idiopathic hypercalcuria	Tuberculosis Neoplasm Cysts Papillary necrosis Hydatid cyst

Calcification within renal substance is a common finding on straight abdominal x-ray. Its distribution, as shown above, may give a guide to its aetiology. Serial films are often useful in assessing effectiveness of treatment (e.g. staghorn) or confirming diagnosis as the lesion enlarges.

Topic 8: Imaging in renal disease

Imaging of the kidney can be used to investigate both static anatomical detail and functional aspects. The three main techniques, ultrasound, radiography and radionucleotide scanning give different information which is often complementary rather than exclusive.

Ultrasound is increasing in popularity with new technology and increased availability. It is a quick and non-invasive method of demonstrating renal size and position and intrarenal lesions such as cysts and tumours, or evidence of obstruction with dilated calyces. It is useful to locate the kidneys prior to biopsy. It may also be used to assess the patency of renal veins in excluding a diagnosis of renal vein thrombosis. Ultrasound is often used as an initial investigation in renal failure before proceeding to more invasive techniques.

Radiography encompasses intravenous urography, retrograde pyelography, renal arteriography, micturating cystography and computerized tomography. Most of these techniques are involved with demonstrating anatomical detail with different degrees of invasiveness and risk. A fair assessment of differential renal function is possible though it can be misleading. An urgent high dose IVU is often the choice investigation in acute renal failure of unknown cause; the aim is to assess the renal size and exclude obstruction. Urography is contraindicated in patients with a history of iodine sensitivity and fine detail cannot be obtained readily when glomerular filtration rate is below 15 ml/minute.

Radionucleotides are increasingly used though several investigations are still research procedures with limited clinical value. Tests of total renal function, using ^{51}chromium EDTA clearance (for GFR) and ^{131}I Hippuran (for effective renal plasma flow) are performed using injection of the isotope and subsequent blood sampling.

Renography using probe counters placed over each kidney, bladder and heart is being replaced by dynamic functional imaging using the gamma camera from which renogram curves can be derived with the use of a computer.

Dynamic imaging is best at showing divided and intrarenal function. It is performed using ^{99m}technetium DTPA, which is filtered by the glomerulus and rapidly excreted. After an intravenous bolus dose rapid sequence imaging shows renal arterial perfusion, whilst subsequent images demonstrate transit through the kidney and excretion into the calyces, pelvis, ureter and bladder. From these images and by selecting areas of parenchyma or pelvis for computer-assisted counting, renogram and elimination curves can be produced. Divided renal and differential intrarenal perfusion can be assessed in experienced units. Renal artery stenosis can be demonstrated and functions of each kidney calculated. Obstruction in the collecting system can be shown by measuring the rate of drainage. Differential diagnosis from a large volume atonic collecting system is achieved by administering frusemide which flushes the normal kidney with washout of isotope but with little effect on the obstructed side (see figure). Space occupying lesions such as cysts or tumours may be demonstrated as either cold or hot areas respectively on the DTPA scan.

In renal transplantation nucleotides have a major role to assess serial renal function and in the differential diagnosis of oligoanuria. In acute tubular necrosis there is good perfusion with no glomerular filtration or excretion whilst in acute rejection there is poor perfusion with no excretion.

Future and as yet experimental technique in imaging include the exciting development of the noninvasive nuclear magnetic resonance (NMR). This will enable the study of dynamic metabolism at the molecular level within particular organs, e.g. ATP → ADP conversion. It will also give static images similar to present computerized tomography pictures representing the distribution of particular ions.

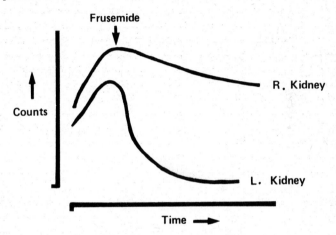

Derived renogram curves from gamma camera scanning using counts from renal pelvis area. Frusemide has enhanced the washout effect in the non-obstructed kidney.

Use of imaging techniques I

Requirement	Ultra-sound	IVU	^{131}I Hippuran ERPF	Technetium DTPA	Renal arteriography	Micturating cystogram
Kidney size	++	++	−	−	++	−
Kidney position	++	++	−	+	++	−
Pelvicalyceal anatomy	−	++	−	−	−	−
Renal calculi	++	++	−	−	−	−
Ureter + bladder anatomy	−	++	−	−	−	−
Ureteric reflux	−	−	−	+	−	++
Bladder emptying	−	++	−	+	−	−
Bladder dynamics	−	−	−	−	−	++
Renal masses (solid/cystic)	++	−	−	−	+	−
Renal blood flow	−	−	++	−	−	−
Renal arteries veins	−	−	−	−	++	−

146

Use of imaging techniques II

Indication	Investigation	Comment
Acute renal failure	High dose IVU Ultrasound ? ^{99}Technetium DTPA	To assess renal size and exclude obstruction. Technetium may be useful to show blood supply to kidney
Chronic renal failure	Ultrasound IVU Retrograde pyelogram	Renal size and shape
Hypertension to exclude renal artery stenosis	^{99}Technetium DTPA Divided renal studies → arteriography	A better screening test than an IVU
Haematuria ? SOL kidney	IVU → (arteriography if indicated) Ultrasound	
Loin pain (to exclude obstruction)	^{99}Technetium DTPA Renogram + diuresis	Better than IVU
Polycystic disease	Ultrasound CT scan	Non-invasive
Recurrent UTI	IVU + micturating cystogram	Looking for an anatomical defect
Renal calculi	IVU Ultrasound	Demonstration of radio-opaque + radiolucent stones

Topic 9: Peritoneal dialysis cannula insertion

Physicians, and even surgeons when not involved in the ritualistic 'scrubbing up', have notoriously bad habits with regard to aseptic techniques. The need for strict adherence to such techniques cannot be emphasized too strongly in the care of dialysis cannulae. This is a good general rule, but has received added impetus recently since many patients who are initially dialysed using the standard 'hard' cannula may subsequently need long-term renal replacement therapy which could be effected by CAPD. This relatively new method of long-term dialysis has as its major complication the risk of peritonitis, and it is possible that a peritoneal cavity which has already been the subject of infection due to careless management in the early stages (i.e. contamination of the temporary dialysis cannula) may be so damaged as to preclude the use of CAPD.

In fact, the aseptic insertion and care of cannulae is relatively straightforward, but the operator must be familiar with the equipment used and should have witnessed at least one insertion before attempting it. A few points are worth stressing. Have the patient lying as flat as possible and ensure that the bladder is empty. The usual place for insertion is one-third the way from umbilicus to pubic symphisis, an area which is relatively avascular. Alternatively either iliac fossa may be used. Avoid areas close to surgical scars, as there may be underlying adherent loops of bowel. Infiltrate skin and subcutaneous tissues down to and including parietal peritoneum. Enter the peritoneal cavity with a yellow 14 gauge needle attached to a syringe containing lignocaine and suck back. If bowel is penetrated, it is unlikely that this small needle will cause the serious problems which may have arisen if the larger trochar and cannula had been introduced directly.

If difficulty is expected, for example because of obliteration of the peritoneal space with adhesions, or the presence of large polycystic kidneys, it is advisable first to run dialysis fluid into the peritoneum through a small cannula. This allows separation of peritoneum and bowel loops and so reduces the risk of perforating a viscus when inserting the larger trochar and cannula.

Before attempting to introduce the trochar and cannula, a small incision, only large enough to accommodate the cannula, should be made with a scalpel blade through skin and subcutaneous tissue.

When entering the peritoneal cavity with needle or trochar, get the patient to tense the abdominal muscles as this facilitates the manoeuvre, which, if the patient has been properly prepared, should require only minimal physical force. Once the cannula is in the peritoneum ensure it is directed towards the posterior pelvic floor; it may be easier to advance if some of the PD fluid is being run in concurrently. The aim is to have the tip of the cannula just anterior to the rectum but without causing pain, therefore advance the cannula until the patient is aware of a sensation in the rectum and then withdraw the cannula 2–3 cm. Once in place, ensure that the metal umbrella is correctly placed, and cut the cannula so that approximately 3 cm remain visible above the skin, pad the surrounding area and connect. It is important to secure the tubing proximal to the connection with the cannula firmly to the patient in order that inadvertent tension on the tube running from the PD fluid bags to the patient is not transmitted directly to the cannula. The first one or two exchanges should be run in and out with no dwell time and each should contain 250 units of heparin per litre — this minimizes the risk of clot formation in the tube, as does flushing the cannula with heparin during insertion.

Checking for faults

Fluid not running:

> Are fluid bags correctly attached?
> Are correct taps open?
> Kinking in the tubing? (especially under the dressing)
> Clots — blood or fibrin in the tube? (Flush, use heparin or streptokinase or insert new cannula)

Abdominal pain:

> Position of cannula? (e.g. too deep causing rectal pain)
> Peritonitis? (cloudy fluid, pyrexia)
> Fluid too hot or cold?
> Hypertonic solution may cause abdominal pain.

Topic 10: Continuous ambulatory peritoneal dialysis (CAPD)

CAPD is a technique of peritoneal dialysis which was developed in America in 1975 using glass solution bottles. In 1977 plastic bags rather than glass bottles were introduced making the technique much more practicable.

In CAPD, dialysis fluid is present within the peritoneal cavity 24 hours a day, seven days a week. The fluid is exchanged by the patient three or four times a day. To perform an exchange, he or she drains out the dialysis fluid into the old bag, then attaches a new bag of dialysis fluid and runs it into the abdomen. This is performed under sterile conditions and takes between 20 and 40 minutes per exchange. A permanent indwelling soft silastic catheter is used with a subcutaneous tunnel to the exit site. It is inserted either under local or general anaesthetic. Each exchange is usually with 2 ℓ of fluid although children use smaller volumes. Patients are normally allowed a free diet, fluid balance being controlled by the use of hypertonic exchanges.

The main advantages of this form of dialysis compared with haemodialysis are that it gives good steady state biochemical and haematological control; allows patients greater mobility; is potentially cheaper; and is particularly suitable for diabetic patients who can utilize the dialysis fluid as a transport medium for intraperitoneal administration of insulin. The main disadvantage is that of peritonitis. In experienced units the frequency is one to two episodes per patient per year. Many of these episodes can be treated as out-patients with intraperitoneal antibiotics, although repeated episodes can lead to debility and loss of peritoneal dialysis surface. Other problems encountered are catheter blockage, abdominal pain with hypertonic solutions, leakage around the catheter, and backache. CAPD may cause or exacerbate abdominal herniae and may also aggravate symptoms of intermittent claudication. Obesity may be a problem with long-term treatment, partly due to the intraperitoneal absorption of dextrose from the dialysis solutions.

CAPD offers an additional and effective form of renal replacement therapy but it must be performed within an integrated renal service offering back up haemodialysis, intermittent peritoneal dialysis and transplantation.

Topic 11: Haemodialysis

Until the relatively recent innovation of CAPD, the mainstay of long-term management of patients with CRF was, and still is in most centres, haemodialysis (HD). Short-term haemodialysis had been possible since the 1940s but repeated vascular access necessary for chronic HD required the development, over 20 years ago, of the Scribner shunt (Teflon tipped silastic tubes inserted into an artery and vein which when not in use are joined by a Teflon connector) and later in 1968 the introduction of the Cimeno—Brescia fistula, where artery and vein, usually at the wrist, are surgically anastomosed which allows repeated vascular access with needles or cannulae inserted into the arterialized vein.

Haemodialysis for acute renal failure, usually for a maximum of 6 weeks, was until recently usually carried out via a Scribner shunt. More recently subclavian cannulation has been used although clotting, wound infection and secondary septicaemia and the risk of pulmonary embolism make this of limited application in the long term.

The mechanics of haemodialysis are in essence quite simple. Blood is removed from the body and pumped through a series of tubes or membranes which separate it from the 'dialysate' fluid which is being sucked in a counter flow direction before the blood is returned to the venous end of the fistula. The dialysate fluid is prepared by warming and mixing fixed volumes of pretreated filtered water with commercially prepared concentrate, so that it contains sodium, potassium and other electrolytes in the desired concentrations. The substances in the blood not present in the dialysate fluid cross the membrane down a concentration gradient. The pore size of the membrane is such that only small molecules can cross and undesirable elements in blood namely products of nitrogen metabolism (urea, etc.) H^+ and K^+ move from blood to dialysate. Larger molecules such as plasma proteins are too large to cross the membrane.

The other major function of the artificial kidney is to remove excess water from the body. This is achieved by altering the pressure between the blood and dialysis fluid (transmembrane pressure) which is the sum of the positive pressure in the blood compartment and the negative pressure generated in the dialysate compartment. By knowing the characteristics of the membrane, the flow rates of blood (usually 200–300 ml/minute) and of dialysate (usually 500 ml/minute) the pressure in each compartment can be preset for the time to be spent on dialysis (usually 4–6 hours three times per week) such that a fairly predictable volume of water, as judged by weight loss, can be removed. This is the ultrafiltration part of the process.

In the UK, unlike most other countries, the accent has been on training patients for home dialysis over a period of about 3 months. They are taught to set up a machine, insert their own needles and connect the tubes up, run their dialyses and disconnect themselves and clean their machines. Once this has been achieved a machine is installed in the patient's home in order to make him or her more independent. Patient survival on home haemodialysis is excellent, greater than 99.5% per month. For various reasons some patients cannot attain this ideal, and need maintenance haemodialysis in hospital, which is more expensive in staff time and facilities.

There are many potential and actual problems encountered however, not least of which is morale. The problems of being dependent on such a system together with disruption of employment and family life, are difficult to imagine. The medical problems — anaemia, abnormal bone metabolism, underlying disease, potential hyperkalaemia and fluid overload resulting from dietary indiscretion are not negligible. Problems related to dialysis itself including haemorrhage and infection must be borne in mind. Some of the gravest problems centre around the fistula itself, clotting of blood and subsequent loss of access, aneurysm formation and risk of high output heart failure particularly in subjects with an already compromised CVS. In most renal units unless there are specific contraindications to transplantation, haemodialysis is performed until a successful graft can be implanted. Nevertheless the majority of haemodialysis patients in the UK return to part or full employment or schooling. This·may in part reflect the limited facilities and, until recently, strict criteria for acceptance on a haemodialysis programme. The period of time on dialysis is variable and for some patients prolonged. There is still reluctance of many doctors to approach the relatives of suitable 'brain dead' patients being kept 'alive' on the life support systems. If these 'lost' kidneys could be salvaged, the quality of life of many patients with CRF could be greatly improved, and release the staff and equipment necessary for treatment of other such patients.

Topic 12: Renal transplantation

Replacement of diseased kidneys with a normal one is the ideal form of therapy. Because of the large functional renal reserve a patient requires only a single transplanted kidney for survival. In the last 25 years successful transplants have become routine and the type of patients deemed suitable has broadened. Though the majority of patients have a primary renal disease such as glomerulonephritis, pyelonephritis or polycystic disease, patients with such systemic diseases as diabetes, amyloid and lupus erythematosus may now be considered. The recipient should have a normal bladder and urethra so that urine from the transplanted kidney can be passed freely. However, transplantation into an ileal loop is possible.

Most transplanted kidneys come from cadavers, though a well-matched donation of one kidney from a living related donor has a higher success rate. The cadaver donors are 'brain dead' but maintained on life support systems. Preferably such a donor should be young, have normal renal function and have 'died' from a primary cerebral tumour or aneurysm, or have been involved in a road traffic accident. Older patients or those with evidence of hypertension or infection are less suitable. Absolute contraindications for donation are evidence of any tumour other than a primary cerebral one and hepatitis. The donor kidneys are removed as rapidly as possible once the circulation has stopped. They are flushed with cold preserving solution and either stored on ice or on a perfusing machine until they can be transplanted. (A perfusing machine pumps cold oxygenated preserving solution through the arterial circulation of the kidney.) Kidneys can be kept by either method for 24 hours before transplantation.

The blood group and HLA tissue type of the donor are matched against a suitable recipient. ABO compatibility is necessary. Opinions vary as to the value of typing for the four HLA A and B antigens and the two DR loci. In broad statistical terms, a fully matched graft will do best, for other degrees of matching the outcome is unpredictable.

The operation involves placing the donor kidney extraperitoneally in the iliac fossa. The donor renal artery is joined either end to end to the internal iliac artery or inserted attached to an aortic patch into one or other iliac artery. The donor renal vein is inserted side to side into the common iliac vein and the ureter implanted in the bladder.

Complications

The transplanted kidney does not always function immediately and may suffer from acute tubular necrosis. Dialysis is then necessary to keep the patient well until the kidney 'opens up'.

All recipients are immunosuppressed to prevent rejection. This is usually with low dose prednisolone (20–30 mg/day) and azathioprine (100–200 mg/day). The prednisolone is reduced slowly to a maintenance of 7.5–10 mg daily. A more recent and promising alternative is the fungal derivative, cyclosporin A. A minor disadvantage is that it is intrinsically though reversibly nephrotoxic, and dosage needs to be adjusted when there is renal dysfunction. Acute rejection episodes, as evidenced by pyrexia, a fall in urine output, a rise in urea and creatinine and a fall in renal clearance of radiolabelled Hippuran usually with a swollen tender kidney are treated with pulse steroid therapy (solumedrone 1 g intravenously per day for 3–5 days). Many patients (including some live donors) have a rejection episode 5 to 7 days after transplantation. Some recipients have three to four such episodes yet still have a successful transplant. Acute rejection is unusual more than 3 months after transplantation. Chronic rejection occurring after 3 months is usually insidious in onset with proteinuria, declining renal function and often hypertension. It does not respond to any treatment. Renal diseases such as a mesangiocapillary glomerulonephritis, Goodpasture's syndrome (anti-GBM disease), oxalosis and amyloid can recur in transplanted kidneys.

Infection in these immunosuppressed patients is a major cause of morbidity and mortality and may be difficult to distinguish from rejection.

Viral infections such as cytomegalovirus (CMV) may be reactivated or transmitted with the transplanted organ causing overt infection 2 weeks to 3 months after transplantation. Herpes simplex frequently causes ulceration in the mouth and fingers and herpes zoster can give encephalitis. Warts occur both on the genital area and on the hands. Bacterial infections occur in the lungs, urinary tract and wound. Pneumocystis carinii is a well recognized cause of atypical pneumonia. Fungal infections are frequent in the mouth with *Candida* and the urinary tract with *Aspergillus* and *Candida*. Immunosuppressed patients with a successful transplant are more at risk from either *de novo* or recurrence of tuberculosis.

Early surgical complications can be due to thrombosis of the renal artery or vein, leakage of urine or the collection of lymphatic fluid in a lymphocyst which may compress the transplanted kidney, its vessels or ureter. Stenosis at the site of the arterial anastomosis can give rise to hypertension though renal vascular bruits are a frequent finding without hypertension.

Complications of long-term steroid therapy (apart from hypertension and Cushingoid features), include avascular necrosis of the femoral head and cataracts. Atypical lymphomas and squamous cell carcinoma of skin have a higher than normal incidence in these immunosuppressed patients.

At present after one year, patient survival exceeds 90% and graft survival is 65–70%. At 5 years for cadaver grafts patient survival is 70% with graft survival 60%. The graft survival is 70–80% for live donor grafts. Most graft losses occur in the first 3 months after transplantation.

Topic 13: Nutrition and renal disease

Diets in renal patients are often inappropriately prescribed and poorly understood. Patients with minimal renal impairment can become malnourished due to severe protein restriction when it is not required and conversely nephrotic patients can be put off by being given too much protein without balanced calorie supplements.

Diets in uraemia

As renal function is lost there is a progressive decline in the kidney's ability to eliminate appropriately water, electrolytes and nitrogenous wastes. Since the amount of these substances to be excreted is determined by intake dietary, therapy is one of the corner stones of patient management. The objective is to maintain the metabolic load within the function of the kidney. Symptoms of uraemia such as nausea, vomiting, anorexia, drowsiness and twitching can be improved by prescribing a diet which is balanced for protein and calories yet affords minimal nitrogen wastage, and so reduces the circulating levels of nitrogen containing catabolites.

Until recently, it was thought that such manoeuvres did not protect residual renal function, but this is now disputed so, in addition to the relief of symptoms, dietary adjustment may prove to be important in delaying the need for renal replacement therapy.

The traditional view is that little protein restriction is needed until nitrogen waste retention causes overt symptoms. The blood urea level is a guide to this, even though urea itself is unlikely to prove a major uraemic toxin. Few uraemic symptoms occur until the blood urea exceeds 30 mmol/ℓ and these disappear if, by dietary means, the blood urea is reduced below this level. However the recent suggestion, cited above, of delayed glomerular loss if nitrogen catabolism is minimized may promote the introduction of selected low protein diets when the GFR is > 25 ml/minute and the blood urea no higher than 12 mmol/ℓ.

The principles of dietary management are straightforward. Protein intake must be reduced, but anabolism ensured by providing that sufficient essential amino acids are taken to achieve maximal anabolism of any other nitrogen in the diet. In practice this means an emphasis on high biological value proteins such as eggs, milk and lean meat or fish, the amino acid content of which resembles most closely that of body proteins. Vegetable proteins are reduced, since with few exceptions they have a very different amino acid composition and nitrogen waste inevitably occurs. An alternative strategy equally effective but with the problem of palatability, is to permit a diet containing varied proteins to taste (but only 20–30 g/day) and supplement this with a mixture of essential amino acids or their keto acid analogues.

With either strategy, adequate non-protein calories (up to 200 kcal/g nitrogen intake) must be taken to ensure nitrogen anabolism and minimize the catabolic effects of gluconeogenesis. To achieve this a variety of protein free foods are available and such calorie boosting agents as Hycal (a starch digest) and Caloreen (a mixture of glucose polymers) are available. Skilled dietetic help is essential in the management of a renal patient.

The amount of sodium and water prescribed in the diet depends

on the ability of the kidneys to excrete or retain sodium and water
and the presence or absence of hypertension and oedema. As the
GFR decreases a greater and greater percentage of the filtered
load in each nephron must be excreted in order to maintain
homeostasis. Rarely, patients with renal failure have a salt losing
state and care must be taken not to induce a negative sodium
balance in these patients as this will lead to worsening of renal function due to a prerenal effect. A normal diet contains approximately
150 mmol sodium while a restriction to 60–70 mmol/day can be
obtained by having 'no added salt' on the table or in cooking. More
severe restrictions of sodium to 20–30 mmol/day require unpalatable tasteless diets with rice as the staple food. It is important to
warn patients to avoid 'salt free' salt as this contains potassium
chloride.

Hyperkalaemia is not usually a problem in chronic renal failure
until the creatinine clearance is less than 10 ml/minute. However
potassium conserving drugs such as spironolactone or triamterene
can induce hyperkalaemia at clearances greater than 10 ml/minute.
Potassium restriction may be achieved by eliminating high
potassium content foods such as chocolate, citrus and dried fruit and
coffee.

Patients on haemodialysis usually require a 50–70 g protein diet
with 500–1000 ml/day fluid restriction depending on residual renal
function and 2500–3000 calories. CAPD patients are often on a free
diet but may require salt and calorie restriction since the dextrose in
the dialysis fluid provides many calories.

Despite the various constraints few patients should be subjected
to severely restricting and potentially undernourishing unpalatable
diets for any length of time.

Dietary management of renal failure: the 'traditional' view (see text)

Serum creatinine (μmol/ℓ)	Serum urea (mmol/ℓ)	Creatinine clearance (ml/min)	Protein diet (g)	Comment
200– 500	5–20	40–15	normal ? 70 g	May need salt restriction
600–1000	20–30	15–5	60–45 g	
1000–1500?	30–50?	5-2	25–30 g	Special bread required

Nephrotic syndrome

Diet and diuretics are the keys to successful management of nephrotic syndrome. Depending on the severity of the illness dietary regimens may vary from a mild protein supplementation to total enteral feeding. A common mistake is to try and give all patients with nephrotic syndrome a 100 g protein diet. This disregards the degree of protein loss or hypoalbuminaemia and often neglects the importance of giving adequate calories to utilize the protein prescribed. If too few calories are taken protein is catabolized to give energy and hence 'lost'.

The following formula is a guide to the amount of protein and calories required:

Protein intake = Urine protein loss (g) + 1 g protein/kg body wt

This then requires 33 kcal as carbohydrate or fat per gram protein. Salt restriction may be necessary to 60 mmol/day, although the use of potent diuretics enables most patients to avoid salt restriction.

Patients with severe nephrotic syndrome may be too ill to eat an adequate diet, in such cases a supplement or the whole diet may be administered continuously in a liquidized form via a fine bore nasogastric tube.

Severely ill acute renal failure patients

These are patients on intensive care units often with multiple organ damage and receiving parenteral nutrition. Debate continues about nitrogen to calorie ratios (150–250 cal/g nitrogen). These patients are often hypercatabolic due to surgery or infection and often have glucose intolerance. Daily dialysis is often required to control urea and electrolytes and to remove sufficient fluid to enable adequate parenteral feeding to be administered. A usual requirement is 2000–4000 cal and 10–25 g nitrogen (1 g nitrogen equals 6 g protein). Calories can be given as 40 or 50% dextrose or as 10 or 20% lipid. In septic patients and those with liver problems lipid should be restricted to one bottle per week, sufficient to supply essential fatty acids. Administration of exogenous insulin is often necessary to prevent hyperglycaemia with the dextrose solutions. Nitrogen is given as amino acid solution containing 10–14 g/ℓ.

Additives are required to maintain metabolic balances. These include phosphate, calcium and trace elements (such as zinc and magnesium) daily, fat soluble vitamins and folic acid twice weekly, vitamin B_{12} weekly and iron monthly.

Topic 14: The face in renal disease

Clinical examination should not be neglected in renal disease because of the relative importance of laboratory investigations in both diagnosis and management. Clues to the diagnosis, e.g. lenticonus, gouty tophi or a lupus rash, may not be apparent from the history. Other signs such as pallor, lemon tinge, band keratopathy, diabetic fundi, acidotic breathing confirm information readily available on routine laboratory tests.

Diagnosis	Case Presentation
Leptospirosis	10
Alport's syndrome	13
Desalination	53
Systemic lupus erythematosus	17
Wegener's granulomatosis	36
Streptococcal glomerulonephritis	16
Disseminated intravascular coagulation	14, 22
Diabetes mellitus	26
Hypertension	3
Gout	7
Nephrotic syndrome	12

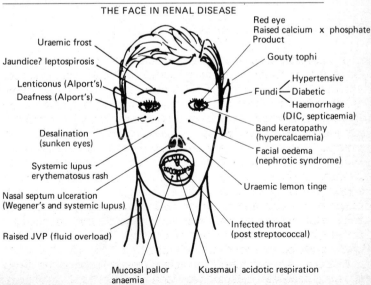

THE FACE IN RENAL DISEASE

Topic 15: Classification of glomerular diseases

It is customary to describe diseases in terms of aetiology, pathology and clinical features, and glomerular disorders should be no exception. However, the aetiology of these conditions is usually unknown, although the demonstration of putative antigens such as HBs Ag in a few patients with membranous nephropathy, and the association of streptococcal sore throat and the subsequent development of diffuse proliferative nephritis suggest that such exogenous (and endogenous) agents are causally related to what are currently designated as the 'immune complex mediated' nephritides. At the present time debate continues as to whether such immune complexes (IC) form in the circulation and are deposited in the kidney or whether the antigen is 'planted' first and subsequently combines with antibody. Furthermore, not all glomerular diseases can be shown to have immune complex involvement — certainly in minimal change nephropathy it does not appear to occur and in focal glomerular sclerosis the aggregation of immune deposits containing complement and antibody may be a secondary event. The role of cellular elements, such as macrophages, in the genesis of glomerular lesions is receiving renewed interest but remains to be determined precisely.

In terms of presentation, the glomerular disorders may be manifest in one of six ways; asymptomatic proteinuria, isolated haematuria, a nephrotic syndrome, a nephritic syndrome, acute renal failure or chronic renal failure, and these clinical syndromes have been used to identify and classify glomerular disorders. The use of percutaneous renal biopsy has enabled a classification to be based primarily on the pathological appearances of the glomeruli, with regard of course to the clinical presentation, and any aetiological relationships.

Pathological interpretation was originally based on light microscopy findings only, but with the advent of immunofluorescent and electron microscope techniques, histological description has become much more sophisticated and certain clinicopathological relationships have been developed, such as the finding of IgA deposits in mesangial proliferative disease associated with recurrent bouts of haematuria, and the demonstration of linear rather than granular deposition of immune deposits in anti-GBM disease.

Unfortunately, there has been, and to some extent still is, a tendency to confuse pathological and clinical descriptions. The best example of this is where a biopsy of crescentic glomerulonephritis is referred to as 'rapidly progressive glomerulonephritis' (RPGN).

While crescentic GN, a pathological description that may or may not be associated with underlying systemic pathology, indeed can progress rapidly with deterioration in renal function this is not invariable and the rate of progress is not accurately assessed microscopically. The term RPGN should be reserved as a clinical description. Similarly, the term minimal change nephropathy has implications with regard to treatment and prognosis. It would be better to leave the pathological description to what is actually seen, e.g. no significant light microscopic changes (NLMC) with or without significant immunofluorescent findings and add subscripts, such as steroid responsive, afterwards. Minimal change nephropathy then is a clinicopathological, not solely histological diagnosis.

Finally, it is still valid to consider these diseases as (i) those where the glomeruli are primarily or solely affected, and (ii) those in which glomerular damage is part of a multisystem disorder. In the latter case, the histological changes may be identical with those of the primary disorders.

Primary glomerular disorders

1. No (significant) Light Microscopic Change (NLMC)
2. Membranous nephropathy
3. Focal and segmental glomerulosclerosis
4. Focal proliferative glomerulonephritis
5. Diffuse proliferative glomerulonephritis
6. Mesangial proliferative glomerulonephritis
7. Mesangiocapillary glomerulonephritis
8. Crescentic glomerulonephritis
9. Unclassified glomerular lesions

Multisystem diseases with glomerular abnormalities

1. Systemic lupus erythematosus
2. Henoch—Schönlein purpura
3. Polyarteritis nodosa
4. Diabetes mellitus
5. Amyloid
6. Scleroderma
7. Rheumatoid arthritis
8. Paraproteinaemias
9. Hypertension

The type and distribution of immunoreactive components and electron dense deposits as well as the clinical setting and response to treatment, and aetiological agent if known, should then be incorporated in a full description of the disorder.

Topic 16: HLA and glomerular disease

The HLA antigens are glycoproteins, the A and B antigens being expressed on most nucleated human cells. They are products of genes located on the short arm or chromosome 6, in an area termed the Major Histocompatibility Complex (MHC).

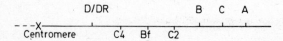

It is interesting to note that components of the complement system, C2, C4 and properdin factor B (Bf) are also coded for in this region.

The A, B and C antigens are detected by lymphocytotoxicity tests on peripheral lymphocytes. D and DR (D related) probably represent the same gene product, but methods used to recognize them are different. The DR determinants are delineated by lymphocytotoxicity testing on fractionated B cells. Mixed lymphocyte culture (MLC) using peripheral lymphocytes allows D specificity to be determined.

Each HLA locus has a number of alleles, approximately 20 for A, 35 for B, 8 for C and 12 for D/DR. Family studies are necessary to determine, in any particular individual, how the observed allelic pattern has been derived from the maternal and paternal haplotypes.

Nephrological interest in the MHC has broadened from the original immunogenetic involvement in tissue typing for cadaver kidney transplantation into suitably matched recipients. Associations are now recognized between some forms of glomerular disease and the possession of particular HLA haplotypes, or specific HLA antigens. In anti-GBM disease for example, 90% of patients have the antigen DR2. Of course it is necessary to relate the observed incidence of an antigen in a disease to the expected incidence in a control population. This is achieved by determining the 'relative risk' of any given individual possessing the incriminated antigen developing such a condition as compared to an individual without that antigen.

Further interest has been generated by the observation that, in some circumstances, the presence or absence of another identifiable gene product coded for within the MHC appears to influence the prognosis. Taking the same example, anti-GBM disease, the presence of HLA B7 heralds a worse prognosis in the HLA DR2 group than does its absence. It is possible that these antigens themselves are in some way responsible for the development and progression of the disease although of course they may simply be a marker for some other pathogenetic gene that is in linkage disequilibrum with DR2 and/or B7.

Some of these glomerular lesions and their HLA associations are given in the following table:

Some glomerular lesions and HLA associations.

	Increased risk associated with	Poor prognosis associated with	Relative risk
Anti-GBM	DR2	B7	27
Membranous GN	DR3	B18/BfF1	12
Minimal change disease	DR7	—	4.7
Mesangial IgA disease	DR4	Bw 35	4
Mesangiocapillary type II (dense deposit)	B7	—	3.7

Topic 17: Complement and glomerular disease

The complement system is involved in the pathogenesis of a number of glomerular diseases. It does not appear to have a major role in minimal change disease, or disorders where there is primarily an infiltrative process going on, such as renal amyloid or diabetes mellitus. The conventionally invoked pathogenetic mechanism in the immune complex diseases (ICD) comprises antigen, either endogenous or exogenous, combining with specific antibody and forming circulating immune complexes (CIC) which become trapped in the glomeruli. There is current controversy about the exact mechanism, and possibly the antigen may be fixed in the glomerulus prior to combination with antibody. Whatever mechanism prevails, though, the end result is glomerular deposition of immunoreactive material which has the ability to further stimulate the immune response by activation of the complement cascade, via the classical or alternate pathways. The complement system has a variety of actions, both in solubilizing IC and in preventing them from becoming too large in the first place and thereby preventing the formation of nephritotoxic CIC. It is worth noting that in a few subjects with deficiencies of early complement components, 'lupus like' syndromes with renal involvement have developed. In these patients it is probable that the failure of complement to interpose in the IC lattice leads to the production of large glomerulopathic complexes. The complement component C3b acts as an 'opsonin' and may coat particles and induce phagocytosis. Some fragments of complement proteins, C3a, C5a, act as chemotactic factors attracting phagocytes. Finally, complete activation of the complement sequence leads to the formation of the 'membrane attack unit' which has the capacity to lyse cell walls of, e.g. invading bacteria.

Immunoglobulins and complement can be detected in various distributions in the glomeruli by immunofluorescent techniques in many glomerular disorders. The type of immunoglobulin detected may have clinical and prognostic significance and potential pathogenetic implications. The nature of the complement components deposited has so far received less attention although the pattern of components deposited has been used to suggest which pathway has been activated. Circulating levels of complement components have to date been of more interest. A low serum C3 level in a nephrotic child suggests that the diagnosis is not minimal change disease; a very low C3 level in an adult might prompt a search for C3 nephritic factor (C3 NeF) and the expectation of mesangiocapillary disease (especially type II dense deposit disease demonstrated histologically). Changes in C4 levels sometimes correlates with disease activity in SLE.

The complement system consists of approximately 19 proteins, comprising about 10% of the serum globulin fraction. There are a variety of components and inhibitors, and activation of the inactive circulating precursors is via a cascade mechanism much like the blood coagulation system.

These reactions are given below in a simplified form. Both pathways eventually lead to the formation of a membrane attack complex which is capable of cell lysis although it is the early steps that appear to be most relevant to glomerular disease.

Classical pathway

The combination of the Fab portion of IgG or IgM with an antigen results in the formation of an immune complex. This results in a modification of the Fc fragment, which is then capable of activating the classical pathway by binding to Clq.

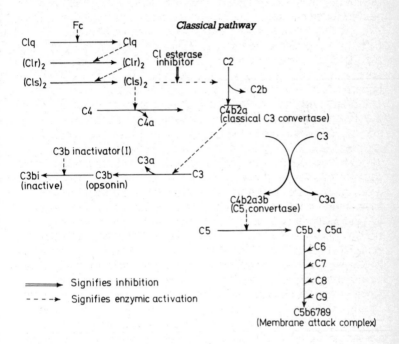

Alternate pathway

The alternate pathway is activated by lipopolysaccharides, many bacteria and viruses, and some IgA aggregates.

The initial step is probably activation of C3, or C3b, in combination with factor B.

Subscript i indicates the molecule to be inactive and as before, dotted lines represent enzymic activation. Once started, this pathway has a positive feedback loop, i.e. the effect of C3bB and C3bBb on C3, which in the absence of inhibitors would rapidly lead to consumption of the relevant components. In some patients with

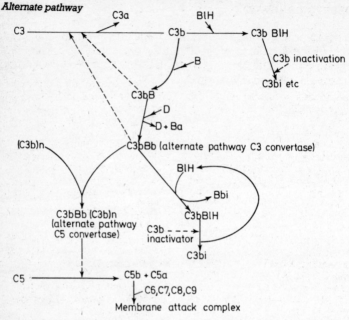

Alternate pathway

mesangiocapillary glomerulonephritis, the presence of an IgG molecule called C3 nephritic factor (C3Nef) induces just such a situation by acting to stabilize alternate pathway C3 convertase and therefore increase C3 consumption.

Index

Abdomen, acute, 16, 17, 40
Acid-base balance, normal, xiii
Acid load test, 88, 138–139
Acidosis, 65
  hypokalaemic, 56
  metabolic, 42, 43
  renal tubular, 88–89, 138
Acute nephritic syndrome (ANS), 34
Acute tubular necrosis (ATN), 11–13, 30
Alkalosis, 65
  hypochloraemic, 115–117
  metabolic, 64, 65, 116–117
Allergic granulomatous disease, 82
Alport's syndrome, 27–29, 102, 157
Aluminium, in dialysis dementia, 87
Aminoaciduria, 83, 84
Amyloid, 11, 45, 68
  A (AA) protein, 45, 68
  in familial Mediterranean fever, 45, 68
  IVU in, 67, 141
  P (SAP) protein, serum, 45, 68
  primary, 45, 66–69
  secondary, 44–46
Analgesic nephropathy, 31–33, 73
  loin pain haematuria, 128
Aneurysms, berry, 3
Angioplasty, percutaneous transluminal, 20
Angiotensin II, 19, 20
  converting enzyme (ACE) inhibitors, 20
  resistance, 65
Antidiuretic hormone (ADH), 114
  in water deprivation test, 139
Anti-GBM disease, 72–75, 161
  HLA in, 74, 161
Antinuclear factor (ANF), 38
Arteries in malignant hypertension, 5, 6
Arteriography, renal, 145
Arteriovenous fistula, 32, 149
Autotransplantation, kidney, 19

Bacterial endocarditis, sub-acute, 29–31
Bartter's syndrome, 63–66
Bence-Jones protein, 9–11, 56
Berger's disease, 35, 61–63, 103

  vs. Henoch–Schönlein syndrome, 126
Bicarbonate infusion, 138
Biopsy, renal,
  percutaneous, 51, 159
Blackwater fever syndrome, 101
Bladder tumour, 89–91
β-Blocking drugs, in pre-eclamptic
    toxaemia, 24
Blood,
  cells, in urine, 130–131
  flow rate, renal, 134
  normal values, xi–xii
  in urinalysis, 130
Blood pressure, in hypertension, 5, 6
Blood transfusion, mis-matched, 48–50
Bronchiectasis, 46

Cadmium nephropathy, 82–85
Calcification of kidney, 143 (see also
    Kidney stone)
  staghorn, 77, 78, 143
Calcium, in hyperparathyroidism, 95
Calcium gluconate, 12
Calcium oxalate stones, 78, 88–89
Calculi, renal, see Kidney stone
CAPD, see Continuous ambulatory
    peritoneal dialysis
Captopril, 109
Carcinoma,
  associated glomerular disease, 122
  of bronchus, 122, 123, 126
Casts, 131–132
  cellular, 132
  granular, 131
  hyaline, 131
  in leptospirosis, 21
  in light chain disease, 10–11
Cerebrovascular accident, 3
Chest x-ray, 140
Colic, renal, (see also Pain)
  in hypernephroma, 110
  in medullary sponge kidney, 75, 76
Complement, 161
  alternate pathway, 163–164
  classical pathway, 163
  components in, 163–164

Complement (*cont.*)
  in Henoch–Schönlein syndrome, 125
  in mesangiocapillary glomerulo-
      nephritis, 92–93
  in post streptococcal glomerulo-
      nephritis, 35, 36
  in SLE, 39
  total haemolytic (THC) activity, 92
Conn's syndrome, 6
Continuous ambulatory peritoneal
    dialysis (CAPD), 148–149
  diet in, 155
  peritonitis, 148
Contraceptive, oral, 127, 128
Copper poisoning, 84
Creatinine clearance (Ccr), 132–134
Cryoglobulinaemia, 106–108
Cyclophosphamide,
  bladder malignancy from, 91
  in minimal change nephropathy, 26
  in Wegener's granulomatosis, 81
Cyclosporin A, 152
Cyst(s), in medullary cystic disease, 4, 77
Cystic diseases, of kidney, 4, 77, 141
Cystinosis, 56
Cystinuria, 77–79
Cystogram, micturating, 145

Deafness, nerve, 27, 28, 103
Dehydration, in hyperviscosity
    syndrome, 112, 113
Demeclocycline, 115
Dense deposit disease (DDD), 91–93,
    161, 162
Desferrioxamine, 87
Diabetes insipidus, 113–115
  central, 114
  -like syndrome, in obstructive
      uropathy, 2
  nephrogenic, 114
  water deprivation/vasopressin test,
    139
Diabetes mellitus, 57–59, 113, 114
  face in, 158
Dialysis, (*see also* Haemodialysis)
  CAPD in diabetic renal failure, 59
  diet in, 155
  dementia, 85–87
  peritoneal, cannula insertion, 146–148
    faults, checks for, 148
Diets,
  in nephrotic syndrome, 155
  in active renal failure, 155–156

  in uraemia, 153–155
Disseminated intravascular coagulation
    (DIC),
  in acute tubular necrosis, 13
  face in, 157
  in incompatible blood transfusion, 49,
    50
  in leptospirosis, 21
  in pre-eclampsia, 23
  in subacute bacterial endocarditis, 30
Diuretics,
  abuse, renal potassium wasting, 64
  thiazide, in diabetes insipidus, 115
Drug(s),
  to avoid, in renal failure, 137
  dosage adjustment requirement,
    136–137
  induced interstitial nephritis, 120–121
  induced lupus, 59–61
  induced nephrotic syndrome, 109
  nephrotoxic, 135
  in renal disease, 134–137
Duodenal obstruction, 117
Dysarthria, 85, 86
Dyspnoea, in renal tuberculosis, 42, 43

Encephalopathy, dialysis, 85–87
Endocarditis, subacute bacterial, 29–31
Epistaxis, 21, 22
Epithelial cells, in urine, 131
Erythrocyte sedimentation rate (ESR),
  17
Escherichia coli in acute prostatitis, 98,
  99
Eye, in Alport's syndrome, 28

Face, in renal disease, 157
Fanconi's syndrome, 55–56
Fat bodies, in urine, 132
Focal segmental glomerulosclerosis
    (FSGS), 15–18, 26, 159
Fundi, in renal disease, 158

Gamma camera scanning, 145
Glomerular basement membrane
    (GBM),
  antibodies, 74, 160, 161
  in mesangiocapillary glomerulo-
    nephritis, 92–93
Glomerular diseases,
  classification, 159–160
  complement and, 161–164
  HLA and, 160–161

in multisystem diseases, 159
primary, 159
Glomerular filtration rate (GFR), 132–134
Glomerulonephritis,
  chronic, IVU of, 142
  chronic lobular proliferative, 92
  crescentic, 73, 159
  immune complex, in malaria, 101
  vs. malignant hypertension, 6
  membranoproliferative, 92
  membranous, 7–9, 109, 142, 161
  mesangial proliferative, 50–52, 103
    in Berger's disease, 62
  mesangiocapillary (MCGN), 91–93,
    161, 162
  neoplasia associated with, 121–123
  post streptococcal, 33–36, 157
  rapidly progressive (RPGN), 158
Glomerulosclerosis, focal, segmental
  (FSGS), 15–18, 26, 159
Glucose, in urinalysis, 128
Glycosuria,
  in cadmium poisoning, 83, 84
  in diabetes mellitus, 57
  in Fanconi syndrome, 56
Gold nephropathy, 108–110
Goodpasture's syndrome, 72–75, 81
Gouty nephropathy, 1, 13–15
Grand mal fits,
  causes, 86
  in dialysis dementia, 86
  in haemolytic uraemic syndrome, 46
  in water intoxication, 53
Granulomatosis, Wegener's, 80–82, 141,
  157

Haematuria, 90
  in Alport's syndrome, 27, 28
  in analgesic nephropathy, 32
  benign familial, 101–103
  in Berger's disease, 61
  in bladder tumour, 90
  causes, 62–63
  in Henoch–Schönlein syndrome, 124,
    125
  in hypernephroma, 111
  imaging techniques in, 145
  loin pain, 126–128
  in malignant hypertension, 5
  painless, causes, 91
  in polycystic disease, 3
  in renal tuberculosis, 42
Haemodialysis (HD), 149–151

vs. CAPD, 148
  dialysis dementia, 85
  dietary restrictions, 155
  at home, 150
  in hyperkalaemia, 12
  problems of, 150
Haemolysis, in blood transfusions, 49–50
Haemolytic uraemic syndrome (HUS),
  46–48
Haemoperfusion, 72
Haemoptysis, 74
Henoch–Schönlein syndrome (HSS),
  123–126
  with nephritis, 73, 74, 123, 125
Hepatic failure, in polycystic disease, 4
[131]Hippuran, 145
HLA antigens, 160–161
  in kidney transplantation, 152, 161
  in membranous nephropathy, 8, 162
  in mesangial IgA disease, 62, 162
  in minimal change nephropathy, 26,
    162
  renal diseases and, 160–162
Hodgkin's disease, 122–123
Hydralazine,
  induced SLE, 60
  in pre-eclamptic toxaemia, 24
Hydronephrosis, 2, 141
Hypercalcaemia, 95, 157
Hypercalciuria, 95
Hypercholesterolaemia, 17
Hyperkalaemia, 12
  dietary restrictions in, 155
  treatment, 12
Hypernephroma, 110–111
  IVU of, 110, 141, 142
Hyperoxaluria,
  primary, 88–89
  secondary, 89
Hyperparathyroidism, 76, 93–95, 105
  chest x-ray, 141
Hypertension,
  essential, 6
  face in, 157
  in Henoch–Schönlein syndrome, 125
  imaging techniques in, 146
  malignant, (accelerated), 5–7
    chest x-ray, 5, 141
    in haemolytic uraemic syndrome,
      47
  in polycystic renal disease, 3, 4
  in pre-eclamptic toxaemia, 23
  in renal artery stenosis, 18–20

Hyperuricaemia, 122
Hyperviscosity syndrome, 111–113
Hypoalbuminuria, 16
Hypochloraemic alkalosis, 115–117
Hypokalaemia,
    causes, 64–65
    in Fanconi syndrome, 56
    in renal tubular acidosis, 137
Hypomagnesaemia, 65, 66
Hyponatraemia, 54, 116, 117
    cause of, 54
Hypotension,
    acute tubular necrosis after, 11, 13
    in incompatible blood transfusion, 49
    postural, 58, 77

Imaging, in renal disease, 143–146
    dynamic, 144
    uses of, 145–146
Immune complex(es) (IC),
    circulating (CIC), 162
    in focal segmental glomerulo-
        sclerosis, 18
    in Henoch–Schönlein syndrome, 125
    mediated nephritides, 158
    in post streptococcal glomerulo-
        nephritis, 35
    in SLE, 38
    in subacute bacterial endocarditis, 30
Immunoglobulin, light chains, 9–11
Immunoglobulin A (IgA),
    in Henoch–Schönlein syndrome, 125
    nephropathy, 61–63, 103, 159
        HLA in, 62, 162
Immunoglobulin M (IgM) monoclonal
    cryoglobulinaemia, 107–108
Immunosuppression, 152
Infection, (see also Urinary tract
    infection)
    acute renal failure, 13, 22, 30
    in renal transplantation, 153
    subacute bacterial endocarditis,
        30–31
Injury, acute renal failure after, 11–13
Interstitital nephritis, 119–121
    causes of, 121
Intravenous urograms (IVUs), 141–143,
    144–146
Ischaemic heart disease, 1

Janeway spots, 30

Kass criteria for urinary tract infection,
    118–119

Kidney,
    autotransplantation, 19
    fetal lobulation, 142
    Kimmelsteil-Wilson, 58
    medullary cystic, 4, 77, 105
    medullary sponge, (see Medullary
        sponge kidney)
    normal IVU of, 142
    polycystic, 3–4, 142
Kidney stones, 76, 88
    calcium oxalate, 78, 88–89
    causes of, 88
    in cystnuria, 77–79
    in hyperoxaluria, 88–89
    in hyperparathyroidism, 94
    imaging techniques, 146
    in medullary sponge kidney, 76, 88
    urate, 14
Kimmelsteil-Wilson kidney, 58
Kussmaul acidotic respiration, 157

Lead poisoning, 84
Leptospirosis, 21–22, 157
Leukaemia, 122, 123
Light chain(s) in Fanconi syndrome, 56
Light chain disease, 9–11
Lipodystrophy, partial (PLD), 92–93
Lithium toxicity, 113, 114, 115
Liver cysts, 4
Lung fibrosis, 71, 72
Lupus, drug-induced, 59–61 (see also
    Systemic lupus erythematosus)
Lymphoma, 122–123
    non-Hodgkin's, 123, 126

Major Histocompatibility Complex
    (MHC), 160
Malaria, 99–101
Medullary cystic disease, 4, 77, 105
Medullary sponge kidney, 4, 75–77, 88
    IVU of, 75, 142
Megaureter, 1–2, 142
Mercury poisoning, 84
Mesangiocapillary glomerulonephritis
    (MCGN), 91–93, 162, 163
Metastases, renal, 122
    cannon ball, 111, 142
Methicillin-induced interstitial nephritis,
    120
Methyldopa, 24
Methysergide, 96, 97
B_2 Microglobulin, 83
Microscopy of urine, 130–132

Minimal change nephropathy (MCN), 24–27, 159, 161
  HLA in, 26, 162
Mixed lymphocyte culture, 161
Multiple myeloma, 10, 56, 68, 112, 141
  hyperviscosity syndrome, 112
  light chain disease, 10
  multiple, 10, 56, 68, 112, 141
  primary amyloidosis, 68
  renal damage in, 10–11
Multisystem diseases, glomerular abnormalities, 160

Neoplasia, associated glomerulo-nephritis, 121–123
Nephrectomy, for hypernephroma, 111
C3 Nephritic factor (C3 NeF), 92, 93, 164, 165
Nephritis,
  hereditary chronic, 28–29
  interstitial, 119–121
  salt-losing, 32
  of SLE, 38
Nephrocalcinosis, 76, 87–89
  in hyperparathyroidism, 94
Nephronophthisis, 105
Nephropathy,
  acute urate, 15
  analgesic, 31–33, 73
  cadmium, 82–85
  diabetic, 58
  gold, 108–110
  gouty, 1, 13–15, 158
  membranous, 7–9, 109, 142
    carcinoma associated with, 122
  minimal change (see Minimal change nephropathy)
Nephrotic syndrome,
  in chronic lymphatic leukaemia, 123
  dietary management, 156
  face in, 157
  Finnish type congenital, 103
  in focal segmental glomerulo-sclerosis, 16
  gold induced, 109
  histopathology, 45
  idiopathic, 8
  malarial, 100
  membranous nephropathy, 7, 8
  in mesangial proliferative glomerulo-nephritis, 52
  in minimal change nephropathy, 26, 156

in pre-eclamptic toxaemia, 23
  in primary amyloidosis, 66–69
  in renal vein thrombosis, 40–41
  in secondary amyloidosis, 45, 46
Neurological disorders,
  in dialysis dementia, 86
  in haemolytic uraemic syndrome, 47
  in water intoxication, 53
Nitrogen waste retention, 155
Normal values, xi–xiii
Nuclear magnetic resonance (NMR), 144
Nutrition and renal disease, 153–156

Obstructive nephropathy, prostate, 2
Oedema,
  in cryoglobulinaemia, 107
  in diabetes mellitus, 57, 58
  in glomerulosclerosis, 16
  in minimal change nephropathy, 24–25
  in neoplasia associated glomerulo-nephritis, 121
  periorbital, 25, 33, 34
  in pre-eclamptic toxaemia, 23
  in renal tuberculosis, 42
  in urinary tract obstruction, 1, 2
Oliguria, 34, 36
Osler–Rendu–Weber syndrome, 128
Osteodystrophy, renal, 103–106
Osteomalacia, 55–56
  cadmium poisoning, 84
'Ouch ouch' disease, 84
Oxalosis, 87–89
Oxytocin, 53–54

Pain,
  abdominal, 16, 17, 40
    in cryoglobulinaemia, 106
    in FSGS, 16, 17
    in peritoneal dialysis, 147
    in renal vein thrombosis, 40
    in secondary amyloidosis, 44, 46
    in severe nephrotic syndrome, 16, 17, 40, 100
  bone, in Fanconi syndrome, 56
  loin,
    in diabetic nephropathy, 57, 58
    haematuria, 126–128
    in hypernephroma, 110
    imaging techniques in, 146
    in medullary sponge kidney, 75, 76
Papillary necrosis, 32–33, 142
Papillomata, bladder, 91

Paraproteinuria, 10, 68, 112
Paraquat poisoning, 70–72
Parathyroid hormone, 95, 105
Partial lipodystrophy (PLD), 92–93
Pelvi-ureteric junction obstruction, 142
Penicillamine, 109
Peritoneal dialysis, 146–148
    CAPD, 147–148
Peritonitis, with CAPD, 149
Periurethral gland inflammation, 119
Phaeochromocytoma, 6
Plasmaphoresis,
    in Goodpasture's syndrome, 74
    in hyperviscosity syndrome, 113
Plasma renin activity (PRA), 19–20
Plasmodium malariae, 101
Pleural effusion, 25, 141
Polyarteritis nodosa, 82
Polycystic renal disease, 3–4, 142
    imaging techniques in, 146
Polycythaemia, 111
Polydipsia, 113, 114
    psychogenic, 114
    test for, 139
Polyuria, 114
    in diabetes insipidus, 114, 115
Post streptococcal glomerulonephritis
    (PSGN), 33–36, 159
Potassium, (see also Hyperkalaemia;
    Hypokalaemia)
    depletion, 64–65
        causes of, 65
    raised, treatment, 12
Prednisolone, in minimal change
    nephropathy, 25–26
Pre-eclamptic toxaemia (PET), 22–24
Pregnancy, in chronic pyelonephritis, 70
Prostacyclin, 48
Prostaglandins, excretion, 66
Prostaglandin synthetase inhibitors, 66
Prostate, obstructive nephropathy, 2
Prostatitis, 97–99
    acute, recurrent, relapsing, 98
Protein,
    restriction, in uraemia, 155
    in urinalysis, 128
Proteinuria,
    in acute abdomen, in nephrotic
        syndrome, 41
    asymptomatic, 50–51
    Bence-Jones, 10, 56
    in Berger's disease, 62

    in cadmium poisoning, 83
    causes, 51–52
    in diabetes mellitus, 57, 58
    in focal segmental glomerulo-
        sclerosis, 16, 17
    in gold nephropathy, 109
    in Henoch–Schönlein syndrome, 124,
        126
    in malignant hypertension, 6
    in mesangiocapillary glomerulo-
        nephritis, 91
    in minimal change nephropathy, 25, 26
    in pre-eclamptic toxaemia, 23
    in renal vein thrombosis, 40–41
Psychosis, in loin pain haematuria, 127
    128
Purpura, thrombotic thrombocytopaenic
    (TTP), 47
Pyelonephritis, 32, 33
    chronic, 69–70
    IVU of, 69, 141

Radiography, 145
Radionucleotides, 145
Rapidly progressive glomerulonephritis
    (RPGN), 159
Rash, purpuric, 123–124
Red blood cells (RBC), in urine, 130
Rejection, of transplanted kidneys,
    152–153
Renal artery stenosis (RAS), 18–20, 146
Renal biopsy, see Biopsy, renal
Renal failure,
    acute,
        in bacterial endocarditis, 31
        dietary regimens in, 153–155
        in Goodpasture's syndrome, 73
        haemodialysis for, 149
        haemolytic uraemic syndrome, 47
        imaging techniques in, 146
        incompatible blood transfusion, 49
        in leptospirosis, 21–22
    in paraquat poisoning, 71
    in severe injury, 11–13
    chronic,
        analgesic nephropathy, 32–33
        imaging techniques in, 146
        salt-losing nephritis with, 32
        serum urate in, 15
        from tuberculosis, 42
    diabetic, 57–59
    dietary management, 153–155

in light chain disease, 10
in polycystic disease, 3, 4
Renal tubular acidosis, 88–89, 138
Renal tubular epithelial (RTE) cells in
urine, 131
Renal vein thrombosis, 17, 40–41, 111
Renin, plasma, activity (PRA), 19, 20
Renography, 145
Respiratory failure,
in bacterial endocarditis, 29, 31
in paraquat poisoning, 71
Reticulocytosis, 47
Retinopathy, 57, 59
Retroperitoneal fibrosis, 95–97
Reversed osmosis, 87
Rheumatoid arthritis, 108–110

Salt-losing nephritis, 32
Scholl's solution, 56, 89
Scribner shunt, 149
Sodium, (see also Hyponatraemia)
in diet in uraemia, 155
loss, in vomiting, 116–117
in normal diet, 155
retention, in urinary obstruction, 2
Sodium bicarbonate, 12
infusion, 138
Staphylococcus aureus, 30, 99
Steroids,
in focal, segmental glomerulosclerosis, 17, 18
in membranous glomerulonephritis, 8
Streptococcal infection, 34
Systemic lupus erythematosus (SLE),
37–39
drug-induced, 59–61
face in, 157

Tamm Horsfall glycoprotein (THG), 131
99mTechnetium DTPA, 144, 145
Thrombosis,
in haemolytic uraemic syndrome, 47
renal vein; 17, 40–41, 111
Thrombotic thrombocytopaenic
purpura (TTP), 47
Transplantation, renal, 151–153
anti-GBM antibodies and, 75, 152
complications, 152–153
donors, 151–152
HLA in, 152, 161
nucleotides in, 145
Tuberculosis, renal, 41–43, 73

chest x-ray, 141
IVU in, 42, 142
Tubular acidosis, renal, 88–89, 138
Tubular dysfunction,
in cadmium poisoning, 83
in Fanconi syndrome, 56
Tubular necrosis, acute (ATN), 11–13, 30

Ultrasound, 143–144, 145
Uraemia,
diets in, 154–155
face in, 157
urea levels in, 154
in urinary tract obstruction, 2
Urate,
nephropathy, 13–15
acute, 15
parenchymal, 14
renal handling of, 14
stones, 14
Ureterovesical reflux, 103
Urethral syndrome, 117–119
Urinalysis, 129
Urinary tract,
infection,
acute prostatitis, 97–99
chronic pyelonephritis after, 69–70
Kass criteria, 118–119
recurrent, imaging techniques in,
145
urethral syndrome, 118
obstruction, 1–2, 142
Urine,
examination of, 129–132
frothy, 15, 16, 44
microscopy of, 130–132
24 hours, normal values, xiv
Urogram, intravenous, see Intravenous
urogram

Vascular anomalies, 128
Vasculitis,
classification, 82
cryoglobulinaemia, 106–108
hypersensitivity, 82
Vasopressin, 114
in water deprivation test, 139
Vertebrae, collapse, 9, 10
Vesicoureteric reflux, 69, 70
Vomiting, hyponatraemia in, 117

Waldenstrom's macroglobulinaemia,
112
Water,
deprivation/vasopressin test, 139
in diet, in uraemia, 154
intoxication, 53–54
loss in vomiting, 117
retention, 2

Wegener's granulomatosis, 80–82, 141,
157
Weil's disease, 21–22
White blood cells (WBC), in urine, 131

Xanthine oxidase inhibitors, 15
X-ray, chest, 140–141